Keto Chaffle R
Cookbook

Quick & Easy Lose Weig
Healthier and Irresistib
Watering Ketogenic Waf
Off Your Day

Chef Adriana A. Ha

with the express written consent from the Publisher. All additional right reserved.

The information in the following pages is broadly considered a truthful and accurate account of facts and as such, any inattention, use, or misuse of the information in question by the reader will render any resulting actions solely under their purview. There are no scenarios in which the publisher or the original author of this work can be in any fashion deemed liable for any hardship or damages that may befall them after undertaking information described herein.

Additionally, the information in the following pages is intended only for informational purposes and should thus be thought of as universal. As befitting its nature, it is presented without assurance regarding its prolonged validity or interim quality. Trademarks that are mentioned are done without written consent and can in no way be considered an endorsement from the trademark holder.

Table of Contents

Introduction

Chaffles (cheddar waffles) are made with two main ingredients: butter and eggs; they can be easily cooked at home. You can eat chaffles for breakfast or snacks. Chaffles are healthy food because they are low in carbs and high in protein. The main ingredient use for making waffles is shredded cheese. The simple ketochaffle is fresh, brilliant, dark in color, crispy, sans sugar, low in carb, and simple to prepare with a waffle maker. You can use small waffle iron or big waffle iron for making chaffles; if you have a small waffle iron, you can pour half the batter into the machine and prepare this and then add the remaining batter. If you have a big iron waffle, you can add the whole batter to your machine and prepare this. Chaffles are preparing in a different size, but it depends on the waffle iron. Chaffles are extremely delicious. If you are on a keto diet, then these waffles will be your favorite. These are unique and creative food and garnish your dining table. You can dress up the waffles in many unique ways. You can add berries, peaches, apples, and bananas to the chaffles. You can eat chaffles as sandwiches. Cut in half and pour butter on it. Make chaffle pizza – add pepperoni, tomatoes, cheese, and your favorite topping. Enjoy dessert chaffles – ice cream, yogurt, and frosting. Add yummy addition in chaffles.

In my cookbook "keto chaffles cookbook," there is a collection of sweet and savory chaffle recipes. You can eat savory chaffles at lunch or dinner. You can eat sweet chaffles at breakfast or as snacks. Chaffles are yummy and delicious food and the favorite food of kids. In my cookbook, I included two chapters, "sweet chaffles" and "savory chaffles." You can choose two savories (one for lunch and one for dinner) and two sweet chaffles (one for breakfast one for dessert/snacks). Chaffles are the perfect keto-friendly food because they are low-carb and high-protein. Make yummy chaffles at home.

Cook chaffles without fear!

How to clean waffle maker:

Tip: 1
Use a damp cloth or paper towel to clean any dirt from the waffle iron.
Tip: 2
Soak up the additional oil drips on the grid plate.
Tip: 3
Wipe the exterior part with a damp cloth.
Tip: 4
Wash the cooking plates in warm soapy water. Wash with water.
Tip: 5
Complete dry the waffle maker before using it
Tip: 6
Always read recipes instructions deeply before start cooking
Tip: 7
Do not submerge the waffle maker in the water.

About this book:

In this cookbook, 50 unique and yummy chaffles recipes are included.

In this chapter – sweet chaffles

Recipes intro – it will represent the whole recipe

Additional Tip – For your guidance –how to garnish the waffles or how to serve

Sweet Chaffle Recipes

Keto Blueberry Chaffles

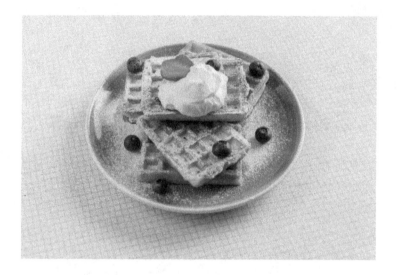

Preparation time: 5 minutes
Cooking time: 7 minutes
Serving: 3

Ingredients:

Beaten egg – 1
Shredded mozzarella cheese – ½ cup
Almond flour – 1 tbsp, optional
Swerve – 1 tbsp
Ground cinnamon – ½ tsp
Vanilla extract – ½ tsp
Frozen blueberries – 2 tbsp

Instructions:

1. Preheat the waffle iron.
2. Break an egg into the bowl. Beat well.
3. Add in vanilla, Swerve cinnamon, almond flour, and mozzarella cheese.
4. Split the mixture into two portions.
5. Add half of the batter into the waffle iron and top with berries. Cook for ten minutes until golden brown.
6. Repeat with the remaining batter.
7. Let cool the waffles.
8. Serve!

Additional Tip:

1. Serve with maple syrup and butter.

Keto chocolate chip chaffle

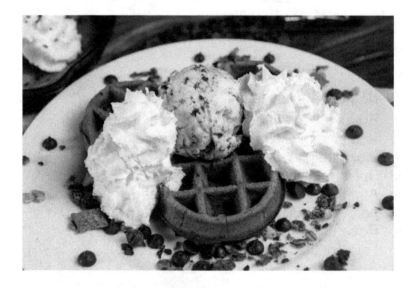

Preparation time: 5 minutes
Cooking time: 8 minutes
Serving: 2

Ingredients:

Egg - 1
Heavy whipping cream – 1 tbsp
Coconut flour – ½ tsp
Monkfruit – ¾ tsp
Baking powder – ¼ tsp
Pinch of salt
Chocolate Chips – 1 tbsp

Instructions:

1. Preheat the waffle maker.
2. Mix all ingredients except the chocolate chips into the bowl. Mix well.
3. Grease the waffle maker. Add half of the batter into the waffle maker.
4. Sprinkle with chocolate chips. Cook for three to four minutes until golden brown.
5. When cooked, remove from the waffle maker. Repeat with remaining waffles. Let sit chaffles for few minutes until crisp.
6. Serve!

Additional Tip:

1. Serve with sugar-free whipped topping or maple syrup if desired.

Keto Cinnamon Roll Chaffles

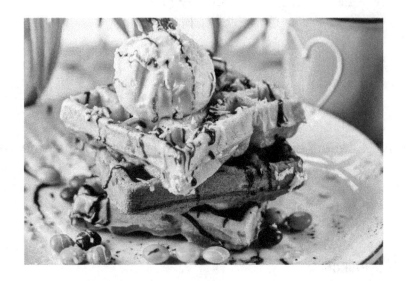

Preparation Time: 5 minutes
Cooking Time: 2 minutes
Serving: 2

Ingredients:

Egg – 1
Shredded mozzarella cheese – ½ cup
Teaspoon vanilla – ½ tsp
Sweetener – 2 tbsp
Ground cinnamon – ½ tsp
Monkfruit Maple Syrup – as needed

Instructions:

1. First, add an egg into the bowl. Beat well. Add remaining ingredients and combine well.
2. Preheat the waffle maker and grease the iron with butter or oil.
3. Pour batter into the waffle maker and close the lid of iron.
4. Cook for two minutes. When cooked, remove from the waffle iron.
5. Let sit chaffles for two to three minutes until firm.
6. Serve and enjoy!

Additional Tip:

1. Serve with butter or maple syrup.

Keto Cream Cheese Chaffle

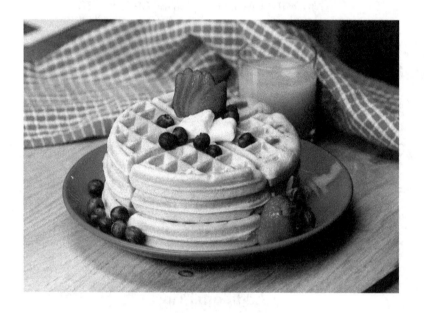

Preparation Time: 3 minutes
Cooking Time: 8 minutes
Servings: 2

Ingredients:

Coconut Flour – 2 tsp
Swerve/Monkfruit – 4 tsp
Baking Powder – ¼ tsp
Egg – 1
Cream Cheese – 1-ounce
Vanilla Extract – ½ tsp

Instructions:

1. Prepare all ingredients. Immerse egg in warm water for three to five minutes.
2. For cream cheese, microwave it for ten to fifteen seconds.
3. Preheat the waffle iron.
4. Add baking powder, Swerve/Monkfruit, and coconut flour into the mixing bowl. Combine well.
5. After that, add vanilla extract, egg, and cream cheese and whisk it well.
6. Add batter into the waffle iron and cook for three to four minutes.

Additional Tip:

1. Serve with favorite topping.

Lemon Ricotta Poppyseed Chaffles

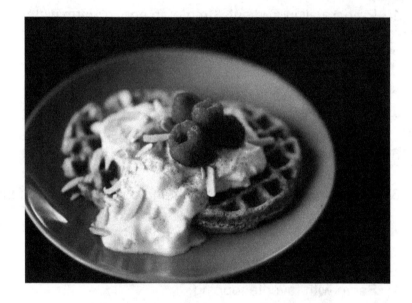

Preparation Time: 2 minutes
Cooking Time: 6 minutes
Serving: 2

Ingredients:

For the chaffle:

One egg – 1
Ground almond flour – 2 tbsp
Part skims ricotta cheese – ¼ cup
Sugar – 1 tsp
Poppy seeds – 1/8 tsp
Fresh lemon zest – ¼ tsp

Optional toppings:

Ricotta cheese
Fresh berries

Instructions:

1. Preheat the waffle iron.
2. Whisk the lemon zest, poppy seeds, sugar, ricotta cheese, egg, and almond flour into the bowl. Combine well.
3. Add half of the mixture into the waffle iron. Close the lid of iron.
4. Cook for two to three minutes. Repeat with the remaining batter.
5. Serve and enjoy!

Additional Tip:

1. Serve with berries and ricotta.

Keto maple pumpkin chaffle

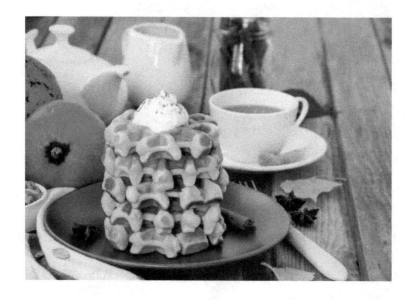

Preparation time: 5 minutes
Cooking time: 16 minutes
Serving: 2

Ingredients:

Eggs – 2
Baking powder – ¾ tsp
Pumpkin puree – 2 tsp
Pumpkin pie spice – ¾ tsp
Heavy whipping cream – 4 tsp
Maple Syrup – 2 tsp
Coconut flour – 1 tsp
Mozzarella cheese – ½ cup, shredded
Vanilla – ½ tsp
Pinch of salt

Instructions:

1. Preheat the waffle maker.
2. Mix all ingredients into the bowl.
3. Pour half of the batter into the preheated waffle iron.
4. Cook for three to four minutes.
5. When cooked, remove from the waffle iron.
6. Serve!

Additional Tip:

1. Serve with keto ice cream or maple syrup.

Delicious Cereal Chaffle Cake

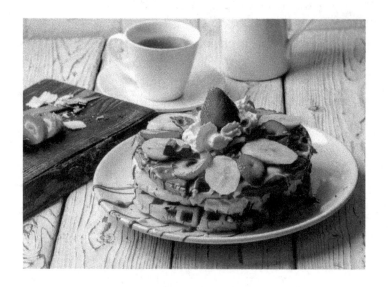

Preparation time: 5 minutes
Cooking time: 3 minutes
Serving: 2

Ingredients:

Egg – 1
Almond flour – 2 tbsp
Coconut flour – ½ tsp
Butter – 1 tbsp, melted
Cream cheese – 1 tbsp
Cereal flavoring – 20 drops
Vanilla extract – ¼ tsp
Baking powder – ¼ tsp
Confectioners' sweetener – 1 tbsp
Xanthan gum – 1/8 tsp

Instructions:

2. Preheat the waffle maker.
3. Combine all ingredients into the bowl. Mix well until creamy and smooth.
4. Let sit batter for few minutes.
5. Add two to three tbsp of batter into the waffle maker.
6. Cook for two and a half minutes.
7. Serve!

Additional Tip:

1. Top with whipped cream.

Yummy Nutella Chaffle

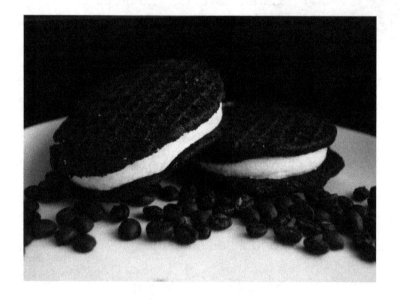

Preparation time: 5 minutes
Cooking time: 6 minutes
Serving: 3

Ingredients:

Dry ingredients:

Hazelnut flour – 3 tbsp
Unsweetened cocoa powder – 2 tbsp
Sweetener – 2 tbsp
Instant coffee – ¼ tsp
Baking powder – ¼ tsp
One pinch sea salt

Wet ingredients:

Egg – 1
Cream cheese – 2 tbsp
Vanilla extract – ½ tsp
Chocolate stevia drops – ¼ tsp

Instructions:

1. Combine the dry ingredients into the food processor. Blend well.
2. Combine the wet ingredients into the food processor. Blend well.
3. Pour half of the batter into the waffle iron. Cook for three minutes.
4. Serve!

Additional Tip:

1. Top with fresh fruits.

Pumpkin Chocolate Chip Chaffles

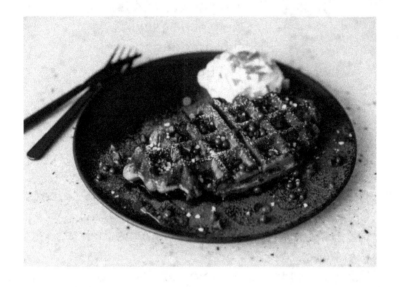

Preparation Time: 4 minutes
Cooking Time: 12 minutes
Servings: 3

Ingredients:

Shredded mozzarella cheese – ½ cup
Pumpkin puree – 4 tsp
Egg – 1
Granulated swerve – 2 tbsp
Pumpkin pie spice – ¼ tsp
Sugar-free chocolate chips – 4 tsp
Almond flour – 1 tbsp

Instructions:

1. Preheat the waffle maker.
2. Combine the egg and pumpkin puree into the bowl.
3. Add in pumpkin spice, swerve, almond flour, and mozzarella cheese and combine well.
4. Add in chocolate chips.
5. Pour half of the batter into the waffle maker. Close the lid.
6. Cook for four minutes.
7. When done, remove from the iron.
8. Serve!

Additional Tip:

1. Serve with whipped cream or swerve confectioners' sweetener

Brownie Chocolate Chaffle

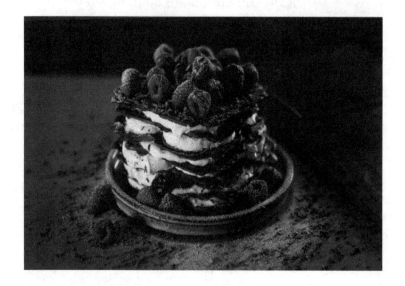

Preparation time: 1 minute
Cooking time: 9 minutes
Serving: 1

Ingredients:

Egg – 1, Whisked
Mozzarella Cheese – 1/3 cup, Shredded
Cocoa Powder – 1 ½ tbsp
Almond Flour – 1 tbsp
Monkfruit Sweetener – 1 tbsp
Vanilla extract – ¼ tsp
Baking Powder – ¼ tsp
Pinch Salt
Heavy Cream – 2 tsp, optional

Instructions:

1. Preheat the waffle iron.
2. Whisk the egg into the mixing bowl. Add dry ingredients and then add cheese and two tsp heavy cream.
3. Add 1/3 of the batter into the waffle maker. Cook for three minutes.
4. Let cool it.
5. Serve!

Additional Tip:

1. Top with chocolate chips.

Cream Cheese and lemon curd Chaffles

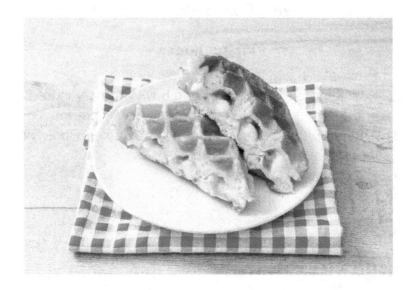

Preparation time: 5 minutes
Cooking time: 4 minutes
Additional time: 40 minutes
Serving: 2

Ingredients:

Keto lemon curd – one batch
Eggs – 3
Cream cheese – 4-ounce, softened
Low-carb sweetener – 1 tbsp
Vanilla extract – 1 tsp
Mozzarella cheese – ¾ cup, shredded
Coconut flour – 3 tbsp
Baking powder – 1 tsp
Salt – 1/3 tsp
Keto whipped cream – optional

Instructions:

1. Prepare the lemon curd and cool it into the fridge.
2. During this, preheat the waffle maker. Let oil the iron.
3. Mix the vanilla, sweetener, cream cheese, and eggs into the bowl and beat well until frothy.
4. Add mozzarella cheese to the egg mixture and beat well. Add dry ingredients to the egg mixture and combine well.
5. Pour batter into the waffle maker. Cook for few minutes.
6. Remove from the iron. Serve!

Additional Tip:

1. Top with whipped cream and lemon curd.

Chocolate Chip Vanilla Chaffles

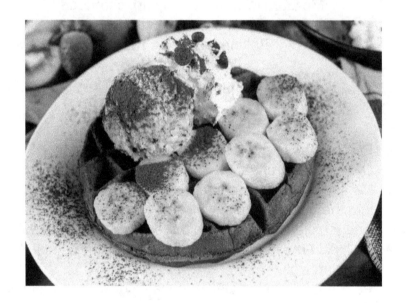

Preparation Time: 1 minute
Cooking Time: 4 minutes
Serving: 2

Ingredients:

Mozzarella cheese – ½ cup, grated, shredded
Egg – 1, medium
Granulated sweetener – 1 tbsp
Vanilla extract – 1 tsp
Almond flour – 2 tbsp
Sugar-free chocolate chips – 1 tbsp

Instructions:

1. Mix all ingredients into the bowl.
2. Preheat the waffle maker. Spray the iron with olive oil.
3. Add half of the batter into the waffle maker.
4. Cook for two to four minutes.
5. Serve!

Additional Tip:

1. Sprinkle with cocoa powder.

Keto ice cream chaffles

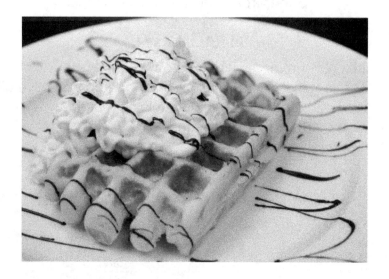

Preparation time: 3 minutes
Cooking time: 12 minutes
Serving: 2

Ingredients:

Eggs – 2
Mozzarella cheese – 1 cup, shredded
Coconut flour – 2 tsp
Baking powder – ½ tsp
Cinnamon – ¼ tsp
Erythritol – 1 tbsp
Keto ice cream – 2 scoops

Instructions:

1. Preheat the waffle maker. Spray the iron with non-stick cooking spray.
2. Combine all ingredients into the bowl.
3. Add chaffle mixture into the waffle maker.
4. Cook for three minutes.
5. Top with keto ice cream.

Additional Tip:

1. Top with whipped cream, berries, and chocolate chips.

Key Lime pie chaffle

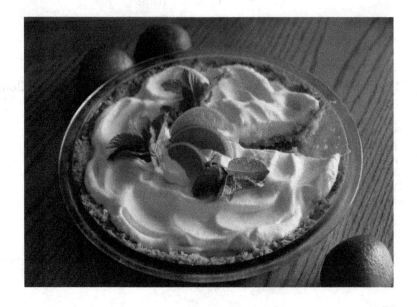

Preparation time: 5 minutes
Cooking time: 4 minutes
Serving: 2

Ingredients:

Key lime pie chaffle ingredients:

Egg – 1

Almond flour – ¼ cup

Cream cheese – 2 tsp

Powdered sweetener swerve or monkfruit – 1 tsp

Lime extract – ½ tsp or Fresh squeezed lime juice – 1 tsp

Baking powder – ½ tsp

Lime zest – ½ tsp

Pinch of salt

Cream cheese lime frosting ingredients:

Cream cheese – 4-ounce, softened

Butter – 4 tbsp

Powdered sweetener swerve or monkfruit – 2 tsp

Lime extract – 1 tsp

Lime zest – ½ tsp

Instructions:

1. Preheat the waffle maker.
2. Mix all chaffle ingredients into the blender and blend on high until creamy and smooth.
3. Cook for three to four minutes until golden brown.
4. For making frosting: Mix all ingredients into the bowl until smooth.
5. Let cool it.
6. Serve!

Additional Tip:

1. Top with butter.

Apple Pie Chaffle

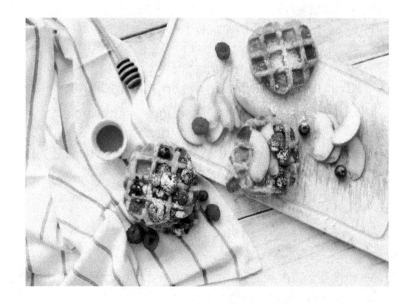

Preparation time: 10 minutes
Cooking time: 10 minutes
Serving: 8

Ingredients:

Eggs – 3
Cheddar cheese – 1-1/2 cups
Butter – 2 tbsp, melted
Gala apples – 4, chopped
Sugar – ¼ cup
Pecans – ¼ cup, chopped
Ground cinnamon – ½ tsp
Whipped topping – ½ cup

Instructions:

1. Preheat the waffle iron.
2. Whisk the eggs into the bowl. Add cheese and combine well.
3. Pour two tbsp cheese mixture into the waffle maker. Close the lid.
4. Cook for three minutes.
5. Repeat with the remaining batter and make seven chaffles.
6. Add butter into the saucepan and cook over a medium flame. Add apples and cook for two minutes.
7. Add cinnamon, nuts, and sugar and combine well. Cover with lid.
8. Cook on low flame for five minutes.
9. Serve!

Additional Tip:

1. Serve with apple mixture.

Blackberry Cream Chaffle

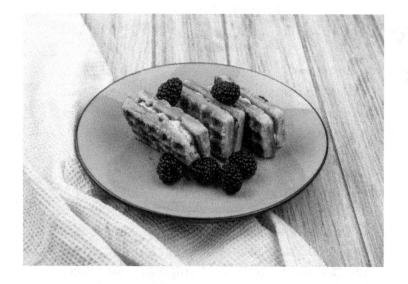

Preparation time: 7 minutes
Cooking time: 15 minutes
Serving: 2

Ingredients:

Cream cheese – 4-ounce, softened
Monk-fruit sweetener – 1 tbsp
Vanilla extract – 1 tsp
Fresh blackberries – ¼ cup, washed and dried
Eggs – 2, big
Coconut flour – 3 tbsp
Baking powder – 1 tsp
Mozzarella shredded cheese – ½ cup

Instructions:

1. Preheat the waffle maker over medium-high heat. Coat the iron with non-stick cooking spray.
2. Add cream cheese into the bowl, and microwave for twenty-five seconds.
3. Add cream cheese into the mixing bowl with vanilla, sweetener, and blackberries and combine with a hand mixer until creamy.
4. Add eggs into another mixing bowl. Whisk baking powder and flour into the small bowl. Add flour mixture and egg mixture into the cream cheese and beat for one minute. Add mozzarella cheese and beat again. Pour ¼ cup of batter to the waffle maker.
5. Cook for three to four minutes until golden brown.
6. Serve!

Additional Tip:

1. Top with blackberries.

Keto Snicker doodle Chaffle

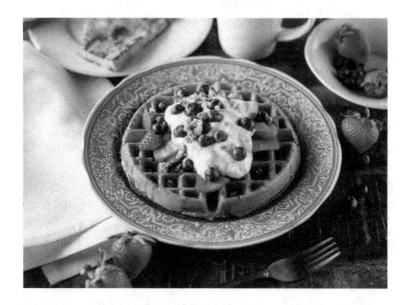

Preparation time: 5 minutes
Cooking time: 10 minutes
Serving: 2

Ingredients:

Egg – 1
Mozzarella Cheese – ½ cup
Almond Flour – 2 tbsp
Lakanto Golden Sweetener – 1 tbsp
Vanilla Extract – ½ tsp
Cinnamon – ¼ tsp
Baking Powder – ½ tsp
Cream of tartar – ¼ tsp, optional

Coating:

Butter – 1 tbsp
Lakanto Classic Sweetener – 2 tbsp
Cinnamon – ½ tsp

Instructions:

1. Preheat the waffle maker.
2. Mix all chaffle ingredients into the bowl.
3. Add half of chaffle mixture into the waffle iron.
4. Cook for three to five minutes.
5. When done, remove chaffle from the waffle maker.
6. Let cool it.
7. Mix sweetener and cinnamon into the bowl.
8. Add melted butter into the oven-safe bowl.
9. Brush the chaffle with butter.

Additional Tip:

1. Sprinkle with cinnamon mixture and sweetener.

Tasty Banana nut chaffle

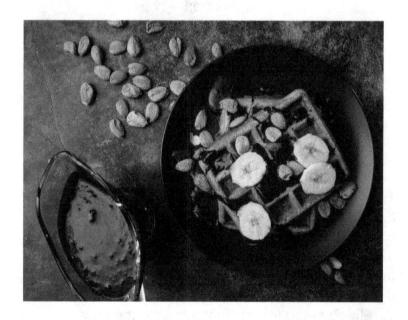

Preparation time: 5 minutes
Cooking time: 4 minutes
Serving: 3

Ingredients:

Egg – 1
Cream cheese – 1 tbsp, Softened
Sugar-free cheesecake pudding – 1 tbsp
Mozzarella cheese – ½ cup
Monkfruit confectioners – 1 tbsp
Vanilla extract – ¼ tsp
Banana extract – ¼ tsp

Optional toppings:

Sugar-free caramel sauce
Pecans

Instructions:

1. Preheat the waffle maker.
2. Whip the egg into the bowl.
3. Add remaining ingredients to the egg and combine well.
4. Pour half of the batter into the waffle maker. Cook for four minutes until golden brown.
5. Serve!

Additional Tip:

1. Top with sliced banana.

Keto Maple Pecan Chaffles

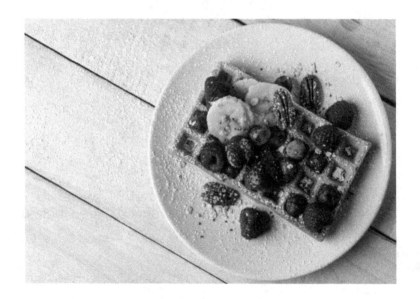

Preparation Time: 5 minutes
Cooking Time: 5 minutes
Servings: 2

Ingredients:

Egg – 1
Mozzarella cheese shredded – ½ cup
Almond flour – ¼ cup
Pecans – 1 tbsp
Monk fruit blend – 1 tbsp
Maple flavoring – 2-3 drops
Coconut oil – no-stick spray

Instructions:

1. Preheat the waffle maker.
2. Add egg into the mixing bowl. Whisk well.
3. Add in maple flavoring, sweetener, pecans, almond flour, and mozzarella cheese and combine well.
4. Spray the iron with coconut oil. Add half of the batter into the waffle iron.
5. Close the lid. Cook for three to four minutes until golden brown.
6. Serve!

Additional Tip:

1. Sprinkle with pecans.

Double Chocolate Chaffles

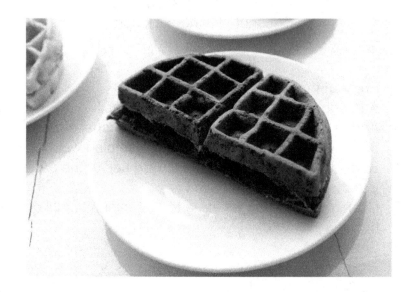

Preparation Time: 3 minutes
Cooking Time: 10 minutes
Servings: 2

Ingredients:

Coconut Flour – 2 tsp
Swerve/Monkfruit – 2 tbsp
Cocoa Powder – 1 tbsp
Baking Powder – ¼ tsp
Egg – 1
Cream Cheese – 1-ounce
Vanilla Extract – ½ tsp
Unsweetened Chocolate Chips – 1 tbsp

Instructions:

1. Prepare all ingredients.
2. Immerse the egg into the warm water for three to five minutes.
3. Microwave the cream cheese for ten to fifteen seconds.
4. Preheat the waffle maker.
5. Add egg into the mixing bowl and beat well.
6. Add baking powder, cocoa powder, Monkfruit/Swerve, and coconut flour into the mixing.
7. When mixed, add vanilla extract, cream cheese, and beaten egg and combine well until smooth.
8. Add ½ of the mixture into the waffle maker.
9. Sprinkle with half tbsp of unsweetened chocolate chips. Close the iron.
10. Cook for four to five minutes.
11. Serve!

Additional Tip:

1. Top with berries and whipped cream.

Carrot Chaffle Cake

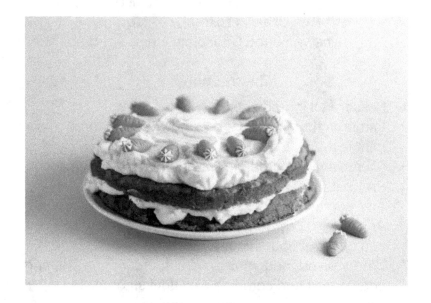

Preparation Time: 5 minutes
Cooking Time: 4 minutes
Servings: 4

Ingredients:
Carrot chaffle cake ingredients:

Carrot shredded – 0.33 cup
Egg – 1
Butter – 1.33 tbsp, melted
Heavy whipping cream – 1.33 tbsp
Almond flour – ½ cup
Walnuts – 0.67 tbsp, chopped
Powdered sweetener – 1.33 tbsp
Cinnamon – 1.33 tsp
Pumpkin spice – 0.67 tsp
Baking powder – 0.67 tsp

Cream Cheese Frosting:

Cream cheese – 2.67-ounce, softened
Powdered sweetener – 0.17 cup
Vanilla extract – 0.67 tsp
Heavy whipping cream – 0.67-1.33 tbsp

Instructions:

1. Combine dry ingredients – walnut pieces, powdered sweetener, baking powder, pumpkin spice, cinnamon, and almond flour.
2. Combine wet ingredients – heavy cream, melted butter, egg, and grated carrot.
3. Add three tbsp batter into the waffle maker. Cook for two to three minutes.
4. Combine frosting ingredients using a hand mixer.
5. Stack waffles and then add frosting between each layer of waffle.
6. Serve!

Additional Tip:

1. Garnish with carrot slices.

Peppermint Mocha Chaffles with Butter-cream Frosting

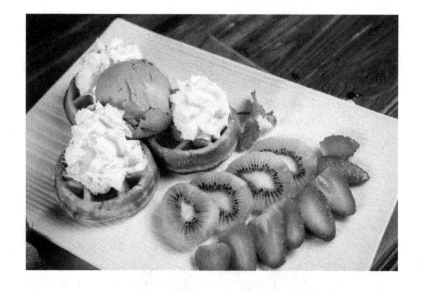

Preparation Time: 5 minutes
Cooking Time: 10 minutes
Servings: 4

Ingredients:

Chaffles:

Egg – 1
Cream cheese – 1-ounce
Melted butter or coconut oil – 1 tbsp
Unsweetened cocoa powder – 1 tbsp
Powdered sweeteners – 2 tbsp
Almond flour – 1 tbsp
Coconut flour – 2 tsp
Baking powder – ¼ tsp
Instant coffee granules – 1 tsp
Vanilla extract – ¼ tsp
Pinch salt

Filling:

Butter – 2 tbsp
Powdered sweeteners -2-3 tbsp, such as Swerve or Lakanto
Vanilla extract – ¼ tsp
Peppermint extract – 1/8 tsp
Optional garnish: sugar-free mints

Instructions:

For the Mocha Chaffles:

1. Preheat the waffle maker.
2. Add all chaffle ingredients into the bowl and beat well.
3. Add two tbsp of batter into the waffle iron and cook for four minutes.
4. Let cool it.

For the Butter-cream Frosting:

1. Beat the sweetener and butter into the bowl.
2. Add vanilla extract and heavy cream and beat at high speed for four minutes until fluffy.
3. Scatter frosting over chaffle.

Additional Tip:

1. Garnish with mint.

Keto Mint Cookie Chaffles

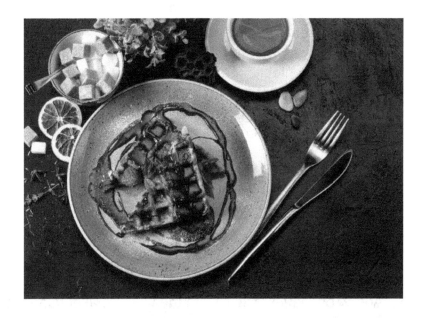

Preparation time: 20 minutes
Cooking time: 2 minutes
Serving: 2

Ingredients:

For the chaffle:

Shredded mozzarella cheese – 1 cup
Eggs – 2, big
Swerve confectioners' sugar substitute – 3 tbsp
Unsweetened cocoa powder – 2 tbsp

For the filling:

Cream cheese – 6-ounce, softened
Almond flour – ½ cup
Swerve confectioners' sugar substitute – ¼ cup
Unsweetened cocoa powder – 2 tbsp
Vanilla extract – ½ tsp
Peppermint extract – 1 tsp

For the chocolate drizzle:

Baking chips – 3 tbsp
Coconut oil – 1 tbsp

Instructions:

1. Preheat the waffle maker.
2. Whisk all chaffle ingredients into the mixing bowl.
3. Add ¼ of chaffle mixture into the waffle maker. Cook for two to four minutes.
4. Remove the chaffle from the iron.
5. Mix all filling ingredients and beat at high speed until smooth.
6. Add coconut oil and chocolate chip into the oven-safe bowl. Melt it for a half-minute.
7. Stack the chaffles and top with filling.

Additional Tip:

1. Drizzle with chocolate.

Avocado Toast Chaffle

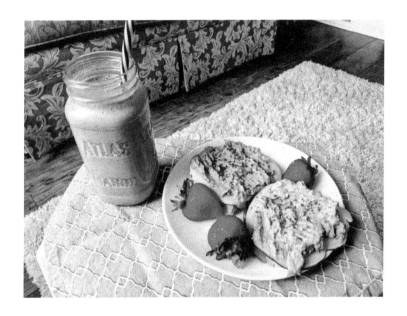

Preparation Time: 3 minutes
Cooking Time: 8 minutes
Servings: 2

Ingredients:

Avocado – ½
Lemon Juice – ½ tsp
Salt – 1/8 tsp
Black Pepper – 1/8 tsp
Egg – 1
Shredded Cheese – ½ cup

Instructions:

2. Prepare all ingredients.
3. Next, peel and slice the avocado and add it to the bowl.
4. Add black pepper, salt, and lemon juice into the bowl. Mash with a fork and mix well. Keep it aside.
5. Preheat the waffle maker.
6. Next, beat the egg into the mixing bowl.
7. Add 1/8 cup of cheese to the waffle maker. Then, add egg mixture. Top with cheese and close the iron. Cook for three to four minutes.
8. Let cool it.

Additional Tip:

1. Top with avocado mixture.

Keto Peanut Butter Chaffle

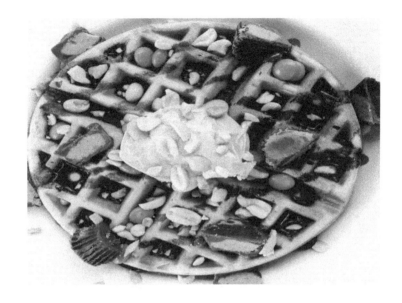

Preparation Time: 3 minutes
Cooking Time: 8 minutes
Servings: 2

Ingredients:

Egg – 1
Mozzarella cheese – 1/3 cup
Monkfruit – 1 tbsp
Peanut butter or nut butter – 2 tbsp
Vanilla extract – 1 tsp

Instructions:

1. Preheat the waffle maker.
2. Next, whisk the vanilla, peanut butter, monk fruit, mozzarella cheese, and egg.
3. Add chaffle mixture into the waffle maker. Close the iron.
4. Cook for three to five minutes until golden brown.
5. Let cool and serve!

Additional Tip:

1. Top with peanuts.

Keto Blueberry chaffles

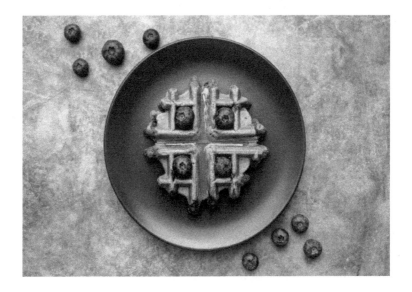

Preparation Time: 15 minutes
Cooking Time: 6 minutes
Servings: 2

Ingredients:
Blueberry chaffles:
Eggs – 4
Shredded mozzarella cheese – 240 ml
Coconut flour – 1 tbsp
Vanilla extract – 1 tsp
Fresh blueberries – 140ml
Serving:
Heavy whipping cream – 120ml
Fresh blueberries – 270ml

Instructions:
1. Preheat the waffle maker.
2. Add all ingredients into the mixing bowl. Beat well.
3. Let rest for five minutes.
4. Grease the waffle iron. Pour the batter into the waffle iron and close the iron.
5. Cook for six minutes.
6. Serve!

Additional Tip:
1. Serve with blueberries and heavy whipping cream.

Keto Lemon Chaffle

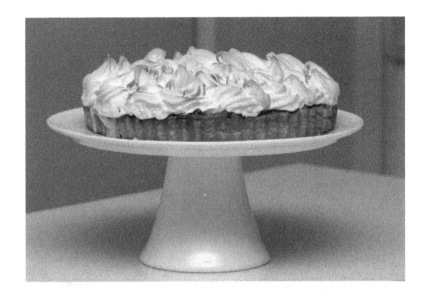

Preparation Time: 5 minutes
Cooking Time: 4 minutes
Servings: 2

Ingredients:
Chaffle cake:

Cream cheese – 2-ounce, softened
Eggs – 2
Butter – 2 tsp, melted
Coconut flour – 2 tbsp
Monkfruit powdered confectioners blend – 1 tsp
Baking powder – 1 tsp
Lemon extract – ½ tsp
Cake batter extract – 20 drops
Chaffle Frosting:

Heavy whipping cream – ½ cup
Monk fruit powdered confectioners blend – 1 tbsp
Lemon extract – ¼ tsp
Optional:

Lemon – peeled

Instructions:

1. Preheat the waffle maker.
2. Add all ingredients into the chaffle cake into the blender. Combine well.
3. Add batter into the waffle iron and cook it.
4. While chaffle is cooking, prepare the frosting.
5. Add chaffle frosting ingredients into the bowl.
6. Mix well.
7. When chaffle is cooled, top with frosting.

Additional Tip:

1. Top with peel lemon.

Keto Birthday Cake Chaffle

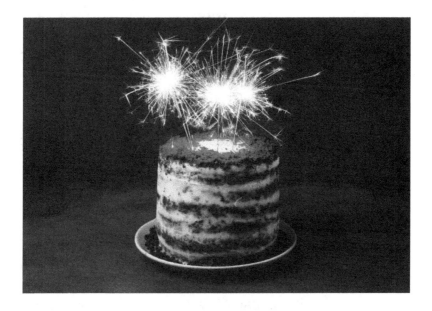

Preparation Time: 15 minutes
Cooking Time: 6 minutes
Servings: 2

Ingredients:

Chaffle cake ingredients:

Eggs – 2
Almond flour – ¼ cup
Coconut flour – 1 tsp
Melted butter – 2 tbsp
Cream cheese – 2 tbsp
Cake batter extract – 1 tsp
Vanilla extract – ½ tsp
Baking powder – ½ tsp
Swerve confectioners' sweetener or monkfruit – 2 tbsp
Xanthan powder – ¼ tsp

Whipped Cream Vanilla Frosting Ingredients:

Heavy whipping cream – ½ cup
Swerve confectioner's sweetener or monkfruit – 2 tbsp
Vanilla extract – ½ tsp

Instructions:

1. Preheat the waffle maker.
2. Add all chaffle cake ingredients into the blender and blend on high until smooth and creamy. Let rest for few minutes.
3. Pour two to three tbsp of batter into the waffle maker. Cook for two to three minutes.
4. **Prepare whipped cream vanilla frosting:** Add all ingredients and combine with a hand mixer.
5. Let cool the chaffle cake.
6. Top with frosting. Serve!

Additional Tip:

1. Sprinkle with sliced fruits.

Banana Pudding Chaffle Cake

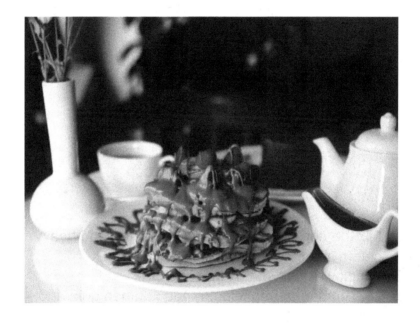

Preparation Time: 5 minutes
Cooking Time: 6 minutes
Servings: 2

Ingredients:

Pudding ingredients:

Egg yolk – 1, big
Heavy whipping cream – ½ cup
Powdered sweetener – 3 tbsp
Xanthan gum – 1/4 – ½ tsp
Banana extract – ½ tsp

Banana chaffle ingredients:

Cream cheese – 1-ounce, softened
Mozzarella cheese –1/4 cup, shredded
Egg – 1, beaten
Banana extract – 1 tsp
Sweetener – 2 tbsp
Baking powder – 1 tsp
Almond flour – 4 tbsp

Instructions:

1. Mix the egg yolk, powdered sweetener, and heavy cream into the saucepan.
2. Whisk well until the mixture is thick.
3. Let simmer for one minute. Add xanthan gum and whisk it again.
4. Remove from the flame, and then add banana extract and a pinch of salt. Stir well. Transfer it to the dish and cover it with plastic wrap.
5. Pour batter into the preheated waffle maker. Close the lid.
6. Cook for three minutes. Serve!

Additional Tip:

1. Top with sliced bananas.

Keto Oreo Chaffles

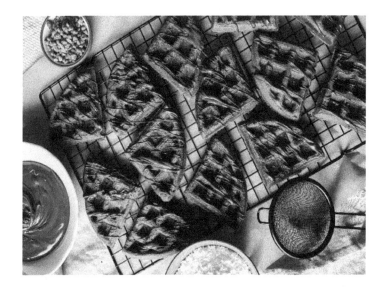

Preparation time: 2 minutes
Cooking time: 4 minutes
Serving: 2

Ingredients:

Chocolate Chaffle:

Egg – 1
Unsweetened Cocoa – 1 ½ tbsp
Lakanto Monk fruit – 2 tbsp
Heavy Cream – 1 tbsp
Coconut Flour – 1 tsp
Baking Powder – ½ tsp
Vanilla – ½ tsp

Filling:

Whipped Cream

Instructions:

1. Preheat the waffle maker.
2. Mix all chaffle ingredients into the bowl.
3. Pour half of the batter into the waffle iron. Cook for three to five minutes.
4. Remove from the waffle maker.
5. Let rest for few minutes.
6. Top with filling.

Additional Tip:

1. Garnish with Oreo.

White Bread Keto Chaffle

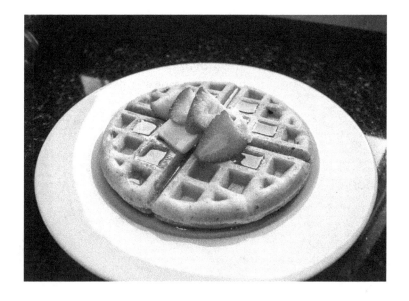

Preparation time: 2 minutes
Cooking time: 8 minutes
Serving: 2

Ingredients:

Egg – 1
Almond Flour – 3 tbsp
Mayonnaise – 1 tbsp
Baking Powder – ¼ tsp
Water – 1 tsp

Instructions:

1. Preheat the waffle maker.
2. Whisk the egg into the bowl. Beat well.
3. Add water, baking powder, mayonnaise, and almond flour.
4. Pour half of the batter into the waffle maker. Close the iron.
5. Let cook for three to five minutes.
6. Serve!

Additional Tip:

1. Serve with butter or jam.

Keto Chaffle Glazed Donut

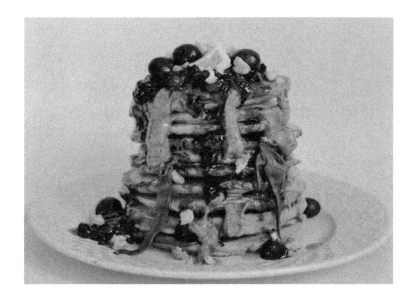

Preparation time: 10 minutes
Cooking time: 5 minutes
Serving: 2

Ingredients:

For the chaffles:

Mozzarella cheese – ½ cup, shredded
Cream Cheese – 1-ounce
Unflavored whey protein isolate – 2 tbsp
Swerve confectioners' sugar substitute – 2 tbsp
Baking powder – ½ tsp
Vanilla extract – ½ tsp
Egg – 1

For the glaze topping:

Heavy whipping cream – 2 tbsp
Swerve confectioners' sugar substitute – 3-4 tbsp
Vanilla extract – ½ tsp

Instructions:

1. Preheat the waffle maker.
2. Mix the cream cheese and mozzarella cheese into the microwave-safe bowl. Cook for a half-minute.
3. Add baking powder, two tbsp Swerve confectioner's sweetener, and whey protein to the cheese mixture and knead with your hands.
4. Add the dough into the mixing bowl. Next, beat vanilla and egg into the mixing bowl until smooth.
5. Pour batter into the waffle maker. Let cook for three to five minutes.
6. Repeat with the remaining batter.
7. Next, beat the ingredients for glaze topping and then add over the chaffles.

Additional Tip:

1. Sprinkle with vanilla extract.

Grilled Blueberry cheese chaffle

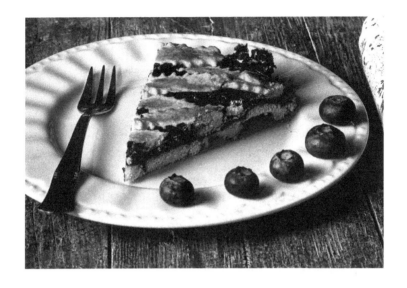

Preparation time: 10 minutes
Cooking time: 5 minutes
Serving: 2

Ingredients:

Blueberry and Brie Grilled Cheese Ingredients:

Blueberry Compote – 1 tbsp
Wisconsin Brie sliced thin – 1-ounce
Butter – 1 tbsp

Chaffle ingredients:

Egg – 1, beaten
Mozzarella – ¼ cup, shredded
Swerve confectioners – 1 tsp
Cream cheese – 1 tbsp, softened
Baking powder – ¼ tsp
Vanilla extract – ½ tsp

Blueberry Compote Ingredients:

Blueberries – 1 cup
Zest of half lemon
Lemon juice – 1 tbsp, freshly squeezed
Swerve Confectioners – 1 tbsp
Xanthan gum – 1/8 tsp
Water – 2 tbsp

Instructions:

Chaffle instructions:

1. Combine all ingredients.
2. Add half of the batter into the waffle maker and cook for two to three minutes.
3. Let cool it. Serve!

Blueberry Compote Instructions:

1. Add all ingredients except xanthan gum into the saucepan and boil for five to ten minutes until thick.
2. Sprinkle with xanthan gum and stir well.
3. Remove from the flame. Let cool it.

Grilled Cheese Instructions:

1. Add butter into the pan and cook over a medium flame.

2. Put brie slice over the chaffle. Top with one tbsp blueberry compote.
3. Place the sandwich into the pan and grill for two minutes until the cheese is melted.
4. Serve!

Additional Tip:

1. Garnish with blueberries.

Keto Strawberry Shortcake Chaffle

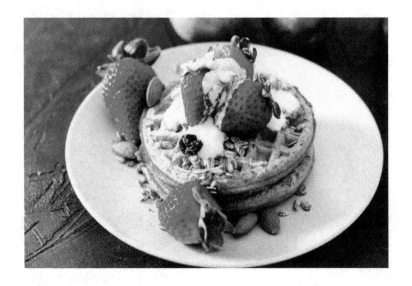

Preparation time: 2 minutes
Cooking time: 4 minutes
Serving: 2

Ingredients:

Egg – 1
Heavy Whipping Cream – 1 tbsp
Coconut Flour – 1 tsp
Lakanto Golden Sweetener – 2 tbsp
Cake Batter Extract – ½ tsp
Baking powder – ¼ tsp

Instructions:

2. Preheat the wafflr maker.
3. Mix all chaffle ingredients into the bowl.
4. Add half of the batter into the waffle iron.
5. Let cook for three to five minutes.
6. Remove and repeat this procedure with 2nd chaffle.
7. Cook for four minutes.
8. Serve!

Additional Tip:

1. Top with whipped cream and strawberries.

French toast chaffle

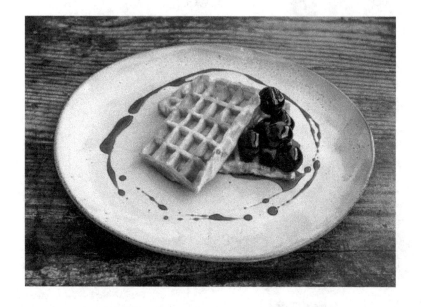

Preparation time: 10 minutes
Cooking time: 5 minutes
Serving: 2

Ingredients:

Egg – 1
Mozzarella Cheese – ½ cup, grated and chopped
Vanilla – 1 tsp
Granulated Sweetener – 1 tsp
Cinnamon – 1 tsp
Almond Flour – 2 tbsp

Instructions:

1. Preheat the waffle maker. Spray the waffle iron with oil.
2. Combine all ingredients.
3. Pour half of the batter into the waffle maker. Cook for five minutes.

Additional Tip:

1. Top with sugar-free syrup.

Keto gingerbread chaffle

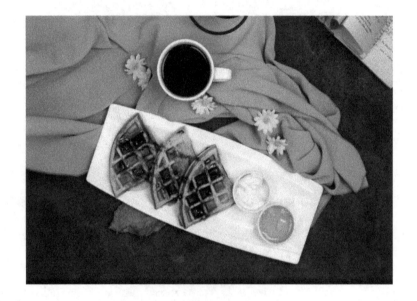

Preparation time: 5 minutes
Cooking time: 5 minutes
Serving: 2

Ingredients:

Mozzarella cheese – ½ cup, grated
Egg – 1
Baking powder – ½ tsp
Erythritol powdered – 1 tsp
Ginger – ½ tsp, ground
Nutmeg – ¼ tsp, ground
Cinnamon – ½ tsp, ground
Cloves – 1/8 tsp, ground
Almond flour – 2 tbsp

Instructions:

1. Preheat the waffle maker.
2. Lightly spray the iron with olive oil.
3. Beat the egg into the bowl.
4. Add erythritol, baking powder, spices, almond flour, and mozzarella cheese and combine well.
5. Add the batter into the waffle maker. Close the iron and cook for five minutes.
6. Serve!

Additional Tip:

1. Serve with cream cheese frosting or whipped cream.

Red Velvet chaffle

Cake

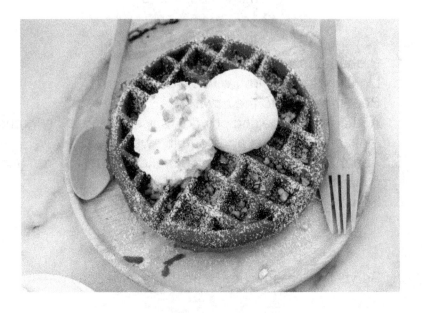

Preparation time: 10 minutes
Cooking time: 5 minutes
Serving: 2

Ingredients:

Dutch Processed Cocoa – 2 tbsp
Monk-fruit Confectioner's – 2 tbsp
Egg – 1
Red food coloring – 2 drops, optional
Baking Powder – ¼ tsp
Heavy whipping cream – 1 tbsp

Frosting ingredients:

Monk-fruit Confectioners – 2 tbsp
Cream Cheese – 2 tbsp, softened
Vanilla – ¼ tsp

Instructions:

1. Whip the egg into the bowl.
2. Add remaining ingredients and combine well until smooth.
3. Pour half of the batter into the waffle maker.
4. Cook for two to three minutes.
5. Add vanilla, cream cheese, and sweetener in another bowl.
6. Combine the frosting until incorporated.
7. Top the waffle cake with frosting.
8. Serve!

Additional Tip:

1. Top with sliced fruits.

Keto Protein chaffle

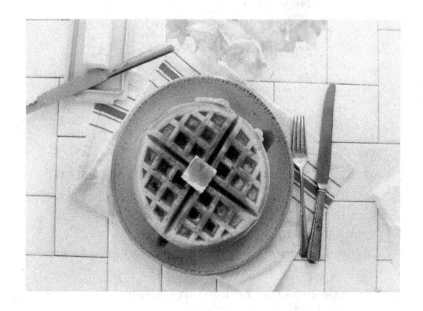

Preparation time: 15 minutes
Cooking time: 15 minutes
Serving: 1

Ingredients:

Protein powder – 1 scoop
Butter – 1 tbsp
Baking powder – ¼ tsp
Egg – 1
Pink Himalayan Salt – ¼ tsp
Liquid – water, almond milk, flax milk

Instructions:

1. Add butter into the mixing bowl.
2. Add the rest of the ingredients and mix well using a fork.
3. Preheat the waffle maker.
4. Add half of the mixture into the waffle iron.
5. Close the lid.

Additional Tip:

1. Serve with maple syrup or butter.

Chocolate cherry chaffles

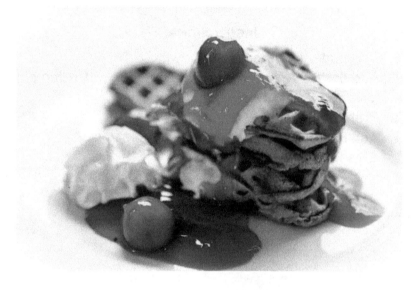

Preparation time: 5 minutes
Cookingtime: 5 minutes
Serving: 1

Ingredients:

Almond flour – 1 tbsp
Cocoa powder – 1 tbsp
Sugar-free sweetener – 1 tbsp
Baking powder – ½ tbsp
Egg – 1
Mozzarella cheese – ½ cup, shredded
Heavy whipping cream – 2 tbsp, whipped
Sugar-free cherry pie filling – 2 tbsp
Chocolate chips – 1

Instructions:

1. Preheat the waffle maker.
2. Mix all dry ingredients into the bowl.
3. Break an egg into the bowl. Combine well.
4. Add cheese and mix well.
5. Add batter into the waffle maker.
6. Cook for five minutes.
7. Serve!

Additional Tip:

1. Top with chocolate chips, cherries, and whipped cream.

Keto cream puff chaffles

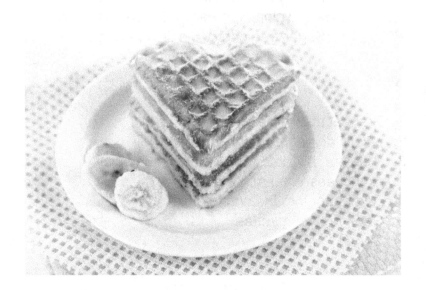

Preparation Time: 15 minutes
Cooking Time: 10 minutes
Serving: 1

Ingredients:

Batter:

Shredded mozzarella cheese or shredded cheddar cheese
– ½ cup
Monk fruit sweetener – 3 tbsp
Egg – 1
Egg white – 1
Heavy whipping cream – 2 tbsp
Coconut flour – 2 tbsp
No-Sugar Butter – 1 tbsp
Vanilla extract – ¼ tsp
Baking powder 1/8 tsp

Filling:

Heavy cream – ¾ cup
Powdered monk fruit sweetener – 1 tbsp + 2 tsp
Vanilla extract – ½ tsp

Instructions:

1. Preheat the waffle maker.
2. Combine the chaffle ingredients into the mixing bowl using an electric mixer. Split the chaffle mixture into six portions.
3. Coat the waffle maker with non-stick cooking spray.
4. Pour one portion of batter into the waffle iron and close the lid.
5. Cook for one minute. Repeat with remaining portions.
6. For the filling: Combine all filling ingredients into the mixing bowl.
7. Top the chaffle with filling.
8. Serve!

Additional Tip:

1. Top with butter.

Keto Coffee Crisp Chaffle

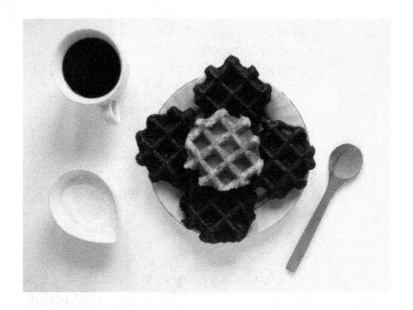

Preparation time: 1 hour
Additional time: 2 hours
Serving: 3

Ingredients:

Chaffles:

Egg – 1
Cream cheese – 1-ounce
Almond flour – 2 tbsp
Granulated sweetener – 1 tbsp
Vanilla extract – 1 tsp
Baking powder – ½ tsp

Coffee Cream Icing:

Heavy whipping cream – 1 tbsp
Instant coffee – 1 heaping tsp
Cocoa powder – 1 tsp
Unsalted butter – ¼ cup, softened
Icing sugar substitute – ¾ cup

Chocolate Glaze:

Heavy cream – ¼ cup
Butter – 1 tbsp
Sugar free chocolate chips – 1/3 cup

Instructions:

1. Preheat the waffle maker.
2. Mix all chaffle ingredients into the bowl. Whisk it well.
3. Add 1/3 batter into the waffle maker. Cook for three minutes.
4. Let cool it.

Coffee icing:

1. Combine the cocoa, instant coffee, and heavy cream into the bowl. Cook for microwave for fifteen seconds.
2. Next, whip butter using an electric mixer until fluffy.
3. Add in a warmed coffee cream mixture and combine well.
4. Add icing sugar substitute and combine well.
5. Cover the chaffle with icing and place it into the refrigerator for one hour.

---

6. **Prepare the chocolate glaze:** Mix the butter and melted cream into the microwave for fifteen seconds. Add in chocolate chips.

Additional Tip:

1. Top with chocolate icing.

Almond Joy Cake Chaffle

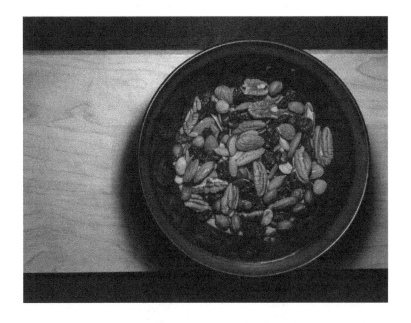

Preparation time: 1 hour
Additional time: 2 hours
Serving: 3

Ingredients:

Chocolate Chaffles:

Egg – 1
Cream cheese – 1-ounce
Almond flour – 1 tbsp
Unsweetened cocoa powder – 1 tbsp
Erythritol sweetener blend – 1 tbsp
Vanilla extract – ½ tsp
Instant coffee powder – ¼ tsp

Coconut Filling:

Coconut oil – 1 ½ tsp, melted
Heavy cream – 1 tbsp
Unsweetened shredded coconut – ¼ cup
Cream cheese – 2-ounce
Confectioner's sweetener – 1 tbsp
Vanilla extract – ¼ tsp
Whole almonds – 14

Instructions:

For the Chaffles:

1. Preheat the waffle maker.
2. Whisk all chaffle ingredients into the bowl.
3. Add half of the batter into the waffle iron.
4. Close the lid. Cook for three to five minutes.
5. Remove from the iron.
6. Let cool it.

For the Filling:

1. Microwave the cream for ten seconds.
2. Add all ingredients into the bowl and combine well.

Assemble:

1. Scatter half of the filling on the chaffle. Add seven almonds on the top of the filling.
2. Serve!

Additional Tip:

1. Garnish with almonds.

Nutter butter chaffles

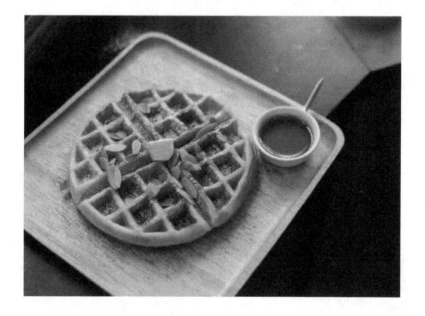

Preparation time: 15 minutes
Cooking time: 14 minutes
Serving: 2

Ingredients:

For the chaffle:

Sugar-free peanut butter powder – 2 tbsp

Maple syrup – 2 tbsp
Egg – 1, beaten
Mozzarella cheese – ¼ cup, grated
Baking powder – ¼ tsp
Peanut butter extract – ¼ tsp
Cream cheese – 1 tbsp, soften
Almond butter – ¼ tsp

For the frosting:

Maple syrup – ½ cup
Vanilla extract – ½ tsp
Almond milk – 3 tbsp
Peanut butter – 1 cup
Almond flour – ½ cup

Instructions:

1. Preheat the waffle maker.
2. Combine all ingredients into the mixing bowl.
3. Pour half of the batter into the waffle maker.
4. Close the lid. Cook for six to seven minutes.
5. Remove from the waffle maker. Keep it aside.
6. For making frosting: Add almond flour into the saucepan and cook for medium flame until golden brown.
7. Transfer the almond flour to the blender. Top with frosting ingredients and blend well.
8. Top frosting over the chaffles.
9. Serve!

Additional Tip:

1. Serve with butter or maple syrup.

Special Bagels chaffles

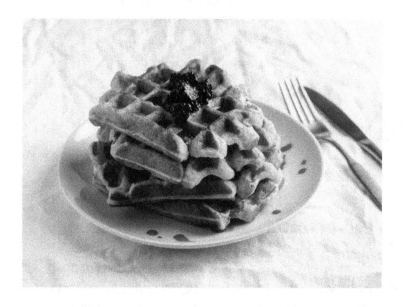

Preparation time: 10 minutes
Cooking time: 28 minutes
Serving: 4

Ingredients:

Egg – 1, beaten
Parmesan cheese – ½ cup
Bagel seasoning – 1 tsp

Instructions:

1. Preheat the waffle maker.
2. Mix all ingredients into the mixing bowl.
3. Pour half of the batter into the waffle maker and close the lid.
4. Add into the serving dish.
5. Serve!

Additional Tip:

1. Top with cheese.

Mixed berries-vanilla chaffles

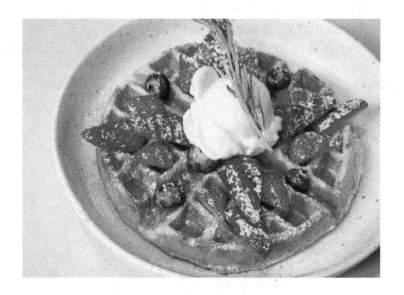

Preparation time: 10 minutes
Cooking time: 28 minutes
Serving: 4

Ingredients:

Egg – 1, beaten
Mozzarella cheese – ½ cup, grated
Cream cheese – 1 tbsp, softened
Maple syrup – 1 tbsp, sugar-free
Strawberries – 2, sliced
Raspberries – 2, sliced
Blackberry extract – ¼ tsp
Vanilla extract – ¼ tsp
Plain yogurt – ½ cup, for serving

Instructions:

1. Preheat the waffle maker.
2. Combine all ingredients into the mixing bowl except yogurt.
3. Grease the iron with cooking spray.
4. Pour half of the batter into the waffle iron and close the iron.
5. Cook for seven minutes until crispy.
6. Top with yogurt.
7. Serve!

Additional Tip:

1. Garnish with berries.

Protein vanilla chaffle sticks

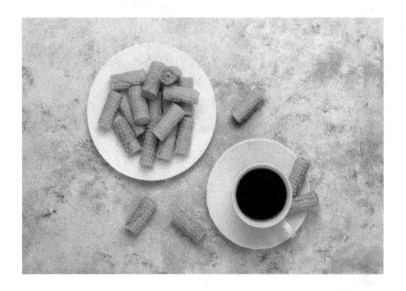

Preparation time: 15 minutes
Cooking time: 14 minutes
Serving: 2

Ingredients:

Vanilla extract – ½ tsp
Erythritol – 1 tbsp
Eggs – 2, beaten
Mozzarella cheese – 1 cup, grated
Protein powder – ½ scoop

Instructions:

1. Preheat the waffle maker.
2. Combine vanilla extract, erythritol, mozzarella cheese, eggs, and protein powder into the mixing bowl.
3. Pour half of the batter into the waffle maker. Close the lid.
4. Cook for seven minutes until crispy.
5. Remove from the waffle maker.
6. Slice each chaffle into four sticks.
7. Serve!

Additional Tip:

1. Top with vanilla extract.

Raspberry-yogurt chaffle

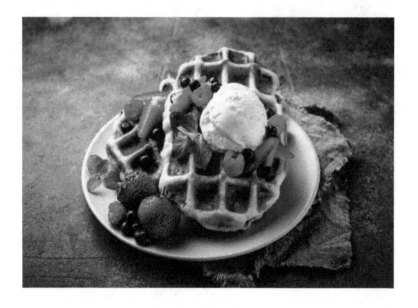

Preparation time: 10 minutes
Cooking time: 14 minutes
Serving: 2

Ingredients:

Egg – 1, beaten
Almond flour – 1 tbsp
Mozzarella cheese – ¼ cup, grated
Baking powder – ¼ tsp
Greek yogurt – 1 cup
Fresh raspberries – 1 cup
Chopped almonds – 2 tbsp

Instructions:

1. Preheat the waffle maker. Grease the waffle iron with cooking spray.
2. Whisk all ingredients into the mixing bowl except raspberries and yogurt until smooth.
3. Pour half of the batter into the waffle maker. Cook for six to seven minutes. Keep it aside.

Additional Tip:

1. Top with raspberries and yogurt.

Keto caramel chaffles

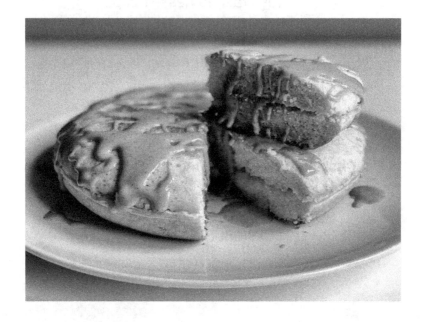

Preparation time: 10 minutes
Cooking time: 15 minutes
Servings: 2

Ingredients:

For the chaffles:

Swerve confectioners' sugar substitute – 1 tbsp
Almond flour – 2 tbsp
Egg – 1
Vanilla extract – ½ tsp
Shredded mozzarella cheese – 1/3 cup

For the caramel sauce:

Butter unsalted – 3 tbsp
Swerve brown sugar substitute – 2 tbsp
Heavy whipping cream – 1/3 cup
Vanilla extract – ½ tsp

Instructions:

1. Preheat the waffle maker.
2. Add two tbsp brown sugar substitute and three tbsp butter into the skillet and cook over a medium flame.
3. Cook the sugar substitute and butter for four to five minutes. Add heavy whipped cream into the mixture and whisk it. Cook on low for ten minutes until caramel sauce is thick.
4. While cooking, combine the ingredients for chaffle into the mixing bowl.
5. Add half of the chaffle mixture into the waffle maker.
6. Cook for three to five minutes.
7. Repeat with remaining chaffles.
8. Turn off the flame and add vanilla extract to the caramel sauce.
9. Add caramel sauce over the chaffle.
10. Serve!

Additional Tip:

1. Top with whipped cream.

Almond flour chaffles

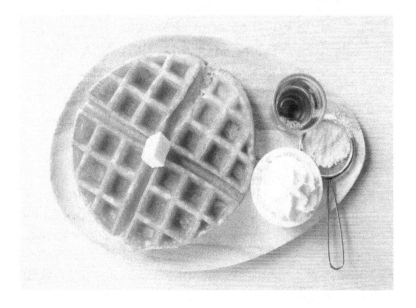

Preparation time: 5 minutes
Cooking time: 15 minutes
Servings: 2

Ingredients:

Egg – 1
Blanched almond flour – 1 tbsp
Baking powder – ¼ tsp
Shredded mozzarella cheese – ½ cup
Cooking spray

Instructions:

1. Whisk the mozzarella cheese, baking powder, almond flour, and egg into the bowl.
2. Preheat the waffle maker.
3. Spray the waffle maker with cooking spray.
4. Add half of the batter into the waffle maker.
5. Close the iron. Cook for three minutes.
6. Let cool for two to three minutes.
7. Serve!

Additional Tip:

1. Sprinkle with almonds.

Psyllium husk chaffles

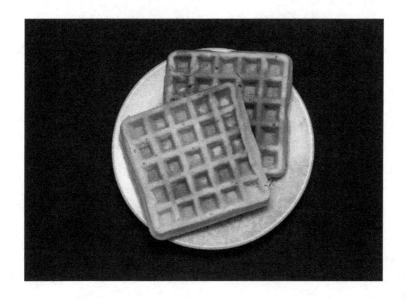

Preparation time: 5 minutes
Cooking time: 4 minutes
Servings: 1

Ingredients:

Mozzarella cheese – 1-ounce, shredded
Cream cheese – 1 tbsp. soften
Psyllium husk powder – 1 tbsp

Instructions:

1. Preheat the waffle maker.
2. Add all ingredients into the blender. Blend until smooth.
3. Add mixture into the waffle maker.
4. Cook for three to four minutes.
5. Serve!

Additional Tip:

1. Top with cream cheese.

Savory Chaffle Recipes

Gruyere and chives chaffles

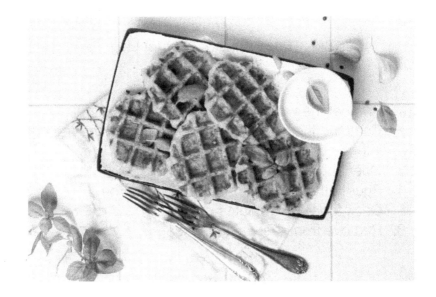

Preparation time: 15 minutes
Cooking time: 14 minutes
Serving: 2

Ingredients:

Eggs – 2, beaten
Gruyere cheese – 1 cup
Cheddar cheese – 2 tbsp
Ground black pepper – 1/8 tsp
Minced fresh chives – 2 tbsp, minced, plus more for garnishing
Fried eggs – 2, for topping

Instructions:

1. Preheat the waffle maker.
2. Combine the chives, black pepper, cheese, and eggs into the bowl.
3. Open the waffle iron.
4. Pour half of the batter into the waffle iron.
5. Cook for seven minutes until crispy.
6. Remove from the waffle maker.

Additional Tip:

1. Top with fried egg.
2. Garnish with chives.

Chicken Quesadilla Chaffle

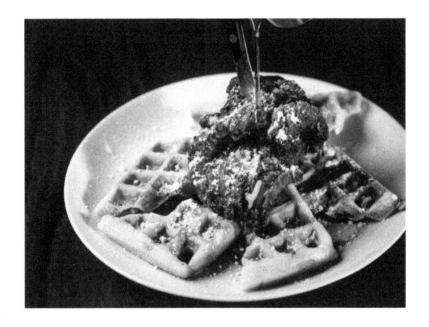

Preparation time: 15 minutes
Cooking time: 14 minutes
Serving: 2

Ingredients:

Egg – 1, beaten
Taco seasoning – ¼ tsp
Cheddar cheese – 1/3 cup
Chopped and cooked chicken – 1/3 cup

Instructions:

1. Preheat the waffle iron.
2. Combine the cheddar cheese, taco seasoning, and eggs into the bowl. Add chicken and mix well.
3. Open the lid. Grease the waffle iron. Pour half of the mixture into the waffle iron.
4. Close the iron and cook for seven minutes until crispy.
5. Remove from the waffle iron.
6. Serve!

Additional Tip:

1. Sprinkle with cilantro.

Scramble egg chaffles

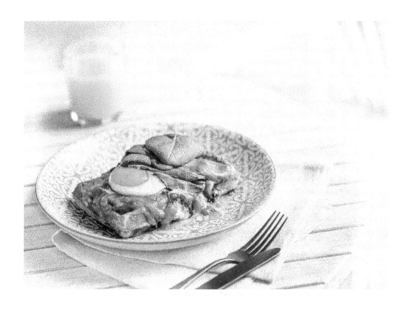

Preparation time: 10 minutes
Cooking time: 7-9 minutes
Serving: 4

Ingredients:

Eggs – 4
Mozzarella cheese – 2 cups
Spring onions – 2, chopped
Pepper and salt – to taste
Garlic powder – ½ tsp, dried
Almond flour – 2 tbsp
Coconut flour – 2 tbsp

Other:

Butter – 2 tbsp
Eggs – 6-8
Pepper and salt – to taste
Italian spice mix – 1 tsp
Olive oil – 1 tsp
Chopped parsley – 1 tbsp

Instructions:

1. Preheat the waffle maker.
2. Break an egg into the bowl. Add grated cheese.
3. Combine well and then add chopped spring onion – season with dried powder, pepper, and salt.
4. Add in almond flour and combine well.
5. Brush the waffle maker with butter, and then add a few batter tbsp into the waffle maker.
6. Close the iron and cook for seven to eight minutes.
7. Prepare the scrambled egg: Whisk the eggs into the bowl for two minutes until frothy.
8. Season with black pepper and salt. Add the Italian spice mix and whisk it well.
9. Add oil into the pan and cook over a medium flame. Add eggs into the pan and cook until set.

Additional Tip:

1. Top with scramble eggs and fresh parsley.

Garlic Bread Chaffle

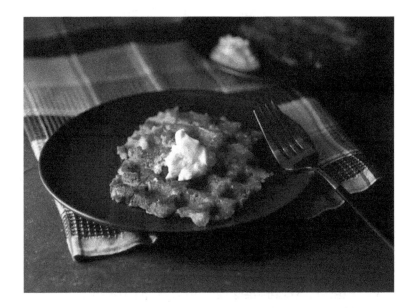

Preparation time: 5 minutes
Cooking time: 10 minutes
Serving: 2

Ingredients:

Egg – 1
Shredded mozzarella – ½ cup
Coconut flour – 1 tsp
Baking powder – ¼ tsp
Garlic powder – ½ tsp
Butter – 1 tbsp, melted
Garlic salt – ¼ tsp
Parmesan cheese – 2 tbsp
Minced parsley – 1 tsp

Instructions:

1. Preheat the waffle maker.
2. Preheat the oven to 375 degrees Fahrenheit.
3. Add garlic powder, baking powder, coconut flour, mozzarella cheese, egg into the mixing bowl. Whisk it well.
4. Add half of chaffle batter into the waffle maker.
5. Cook for three minutes.
6. Place the chaffles on the baking sheet.
7. Mix the garlic, salt, and butter and add over the chaffle.
8. Top with parmesan cheese and place into the oven, and bake for five minutes.

Additional Tip:

1. Sprinkle with fresh parsley.

Tasty Zucchini Chaffles

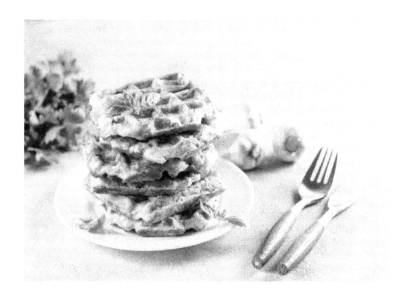

Preparation Time: 10 minutes
Cooking Time: 5 minutes
Serving: 2

Ingredients:

Zucchini – 1 cup, grated
Eggs – 1, beaten
Shredded parmesan cheese – ½ cup
Shredded mozzarella cheese – ¼ cup
Dried Basil – 1 tsp, or fresh basil – ¼ cup, chopped
Kosher Salt – ¾ tsp, divided
Ground Black Pepper – ½ tsp

Instructions:

1. Sprinkle the ¼ tsp salt over zucchini. Wrap the zucchini into the paper towel. Press it.
2. Add egg into the bowl and beat well. Add in pepper, salt, basil, mozzarella cheese, and grated zucchini. Sprinkle with one to two tbsp of shredded parmesan cheese.
3. Scatter ¼ of zucchini mixture and top with one to two tbsp of parmesan cheese and close the iron.
4. Let cook for four to eight minutes.
5. Remove from the waffle maker.

Additional Tip:

1. Garnish with ribbon zucchini.

Keto Cauliflower Chaffles

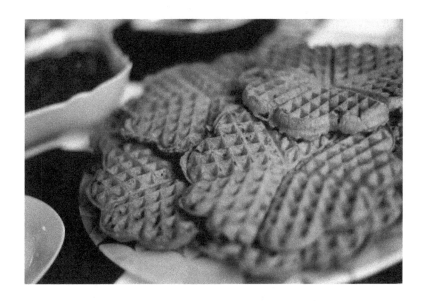

Preparation Time: 5 minutes
Cooking Time: 4 minutes
Servings: 2

Ingredients:

Riced cauliflower – 1 cup
Garlic Powder – ¼ tsp
Ground Black Pepper – ¼ tsp
Italian Seasoning – ½ tsp
Kosher Salt – ¼ tsp
Shredded mozzarella cheese – ½ cup
Egg – 1
Shredded parmesan cheese – ½ cup

Instructions:

1. Add all ingredients into the blender.
2. Sprinkle with 1/8 cup parmesan cheese into the waffle iron.
3. Fill the cauliflower batter into the waffle iron.
4. Top with parmesan cheese and close the iron.
5. Cook for four to five minutes.
6. Serve!

Additional Tip:

1. Serve with mayo.

Keto taco chaffle

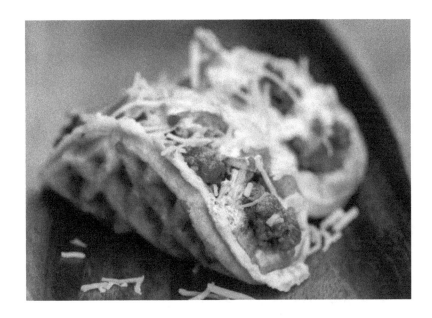

Preparation Time: 5 minutes
Cooking Time: 8 minutes
Servings: 1

Ingredients:

Egg white – 1
Monterey jack cheese – ¼ cup, shredded
Sharp cheddar cheese – ¼ cup, shredded
Water – ¾ tsp
Coconut flour – 1 tsp
Baking powder – ¼ tsp
Chili powder – 1/8 tsp
Pinch of salt

Instructions:

1. Preheat the waffle maker. Grease the waffle iron with oil.
2. Mix all ingredients into the bowl. Close the iron.
3. Pour half of the batter into the waffle iron. Close the iron.
4. Cook for four minutes.
5. Remove and serve!

Additional Tip:

1. Serve with sauce.

Keto chaffle garlic cheesy bread sticks

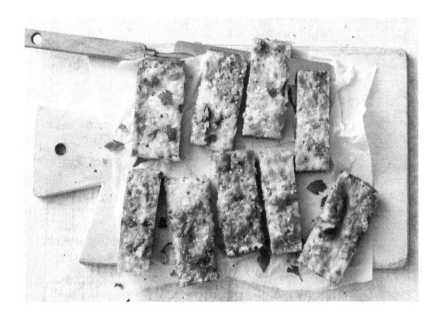

Preparation Time: 3 minutes
Cooking Time: 7 minutes
Servings: 4

Ingredients:

Egg – 1
Mozzarella cheese – ½ cup, grated
Almond flour – 2 tbsp
Garlic powder – ½ tsp
Oregano – ½ tsp
Salt – ½ tsp

Topping:

Butter – 2 tbsp, unsalted softened
Garlic powder – ½ tsp
Mozzarella cheese – ¼ cup, grated

Instructions:

1. Preheat the waffle maker. Grease it with olive oil.
2. Add egg into the bowl. Beat it well.
3. Combine salt, oregano, garlic, powder, almond flour, and mozzarella cheese.
4. Add half of the batter into the waffle maker.
5. Close the lid. Cook for five minutes.
6. Slice into four strips for each chaffle.
7. Place the sticks on the grill. Combine the butter with garlic powder and pour over the sticks.
8. Sprinkle with mozzarella cheese. Place on the grill and cook for two to three minutes.
9. Serve!

Additional Tip:

1. Top with mayo.

keto sausage gravy Chaffle

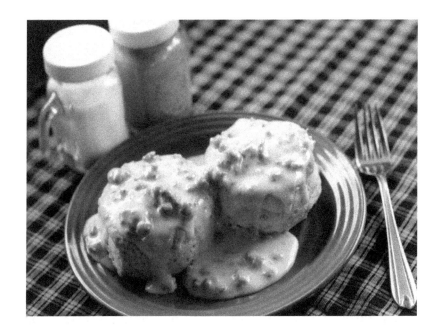

Preparation Time: 5 minutes
Cooking Time: 10 minutes
Servings: 2

Ingredients:

For the Chaffle:

Egg – 1
Mozzarella cheese – ½ cup, grated
Coconut flour – 1 tsp
Water – 1 tsp
Baking powder – ¼ tsp
Pinch of salt

For the Keto Sausage Gravy:

Breakfast sausage – ¼ cup, browned
Chicken broth – 3 tbsp
Heavy whipping cream – 2 tbsp
Cream cheese – 2 tsp, softened
Dash garlic powder
Pepper – to taste
Dash of onion powder

Instructions:

1. Preheat the waffle maker. Grease the iron with cooking spray.
2. Mix all ingredients for chaffle into the bowl. Stir well.
3. Add half of the mixture into the waffle maker. Close the iron. Cook for four minutes.
4. Next, remove chaffle from the waffle maker.
5. Keep it aside.

For the Keto Sausage Gravy:

1. Next, cook one pound breakfast sausage and drain it. Reserve ¼ cup.
2. Wipe additional grease from the skillet and then add ¼ cup browned breakfast sausage and the rest of the ingredients. Boil it and stir well.
3. Decrease the speed of the flame and cook for five to seven minutes.
4. Add xanthan gum and cook until thick.

---

5. Add pepper and salt, and then add keto sausage gravy over the chaffle.
6. Serve!

Additional Tip:

1. Serve with sauce.

Buffalo chicken chaffle

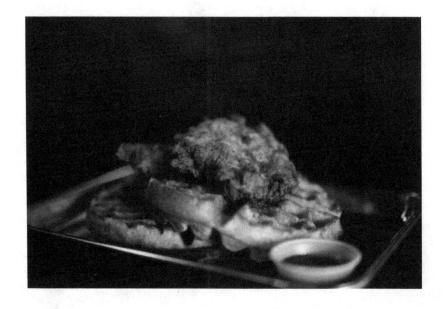

Preparation time: 15 minutes
Cooking time: 4 minutes
Serving: 2

Ingredients:

Almond flour – ¼ cup
Baking powder – 1 tsp
Eggs – 2
Chicken – ½ cup, shredded
Mozzarella cheese – ¼ cup, shredded
Frank's Red Hot Sauce – ¼ cup + 1 tbsp, for topping
Sharp cheddar cheese – ¾ cup, shredded
Feta cheese – ¼ cup, crumbled
Celery – ¼ cup, diced

Instructions:

1. First, whisk the baking powder in the almond flour into the mixing bowl. Keep it aside.
2. Preheat the waffle maker. Spray with low-carb non-stick cooking spray.
3. Add eggs into the bowl and beat well until frothy.
4. Add in hot sauce and beat well. Add in shredded cheese and then mix well. Fold in shredded chicken.
5. Pour chaffle batter into the waffle maker.
6. Cook for four minutes.
7. When done, remove from the iron.

Additional Tip:

1. Top with hot sauce, celery, and feta cheese.

Keto chaffle BLT sandwich

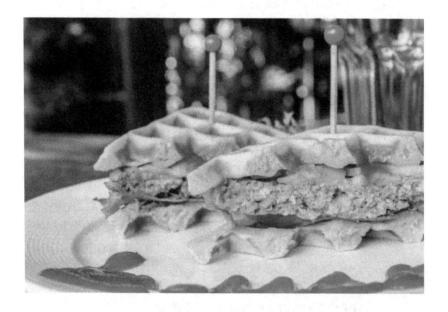

Preparation time: 3 minutes
Cooking time: 10 minutes
Serving: 1

Ingredients:

For the chaffles:

Egg – 1
Cheddar cheese – ½ cup, shredded

For the sandwich:

Bacon – 2 strips
Tomato – 1-2 slices
Lettuce – 2-3 pieces
Mayonnaise – 1 tbsp

Instructions:

1. Preheat the waffle maker.
2. Combine the shredded cheese and egg into the mixing bowl. Stir well.
3. Add half of chaffle mixture into the waffle maker.
4. Cook for three to four minutes until golden brown.
5. Add bacon into the pan and cook over a medium flame. Drain it on the paper towel.
6. Assemble: Stack the sandwich with mayonnaise, tomato, and lettuce.

Additional Tip:

1. Serve with ketchup.

Jalapeno Popper Chaffles

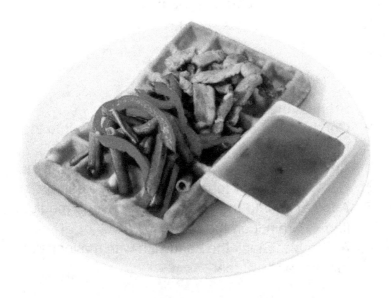

Preparation time: 5 minutes
Cooking time: 5 minutes
Serving: 2

Ingredients:

Egg – 1
Almond flour – 1 tbsp
Shredded cheddar cheese – ½ cup
Softened cream cheese – 1 tbsp
Freshly diced jalapeno – 1/2 tbsp, diced
Crumbled bacon – 2 tbsp
Pinch garlic powder

Instructions:

1. Preheat the waffle maker.
2. Whisk the egg into the bowl. Add remaining ingredients and combine well.
3. Coat the iron with cooking spray. Sprinkle with shredded cheese.
4. Add half of the batter into the waffle maker. Close the iron. Cook for three to five minutes.

Additional Tip:

1. Top with cream cheese.

Salmon tacos chaffle

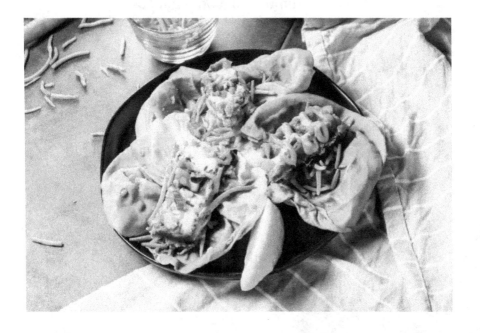

Preparation time: 5 minutes
Cooking time: 5 minutes
Serving: 4

Ingredients:

Salmon – 26-ounce
Almond flour – 1 cup
Eggs – 2
Salt – 1 tsp
Jalapeño – 1, diced
Red onion – 1/2 cup, diced
Green onion – ½ cup, diced
Orange pepper – 1, diced
Garlic – 1 tsp, minced
Dill – 1 tsp
lemon – 1, juiced
Mayo – 2 tbsp
Carrots – 1 cup, matchsticks
Siracha Mayo – 1 tbsp
Greek yogurt – 1 tbsp
Butter lettuce

Instructions:

1. Prepare the ingredients.
2. Drain salmon and dice vegetables.
3. Ass half of green onion, pepper, dill, lemon juice, mayo, garlic, red onion, jalapeno, salt, egg, salmon, and almond flour into the bowl. Combine well.
4. Preheat the waffle maker. Make four to five patties from the mixture.
5. Cook patties for three to four minutes.
6. Slice into strips. Add matchsticks carrot to the butter lettuce tortilla.
7. Add salmon chaffle strips into the middle of butter lettuce.

Additional Tip:

1. Top with sriracha mayo, Greek yogurt, and remaining green onions.

Keto pizza chaffles

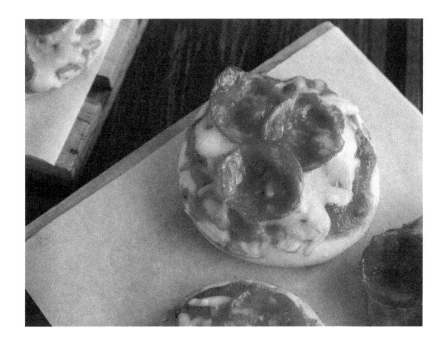

Preparation time: 3 minutes
Cooking time: 7 minutes
Serving: 2

Ingredients:

Chaffle crust:

Egg – 1
Mozzarella cheese – ½ cup, shredded
Italian Herb blend – ½ tsp
Pinch garlic powder

Pizza Toppings:

Tomato sauce – 2 tbsp
Mozzarella cheese – ½ cup, shredded
Pepperoni – 6, optional

Instructions:

1. Preheat the waffle maker.
2. Preheat the oven to 400 degrees Fahrenheit.
3. Combine herbs, garlic, cheese, and egg into the mixing bowl. Stir well.
4. Pour half of the batter into the waffle maker.
5. Cook for three to four minutes until golden brown.
6. Top chaffle crust with pepperoni, cheese, and tomato sauce.
7. Place on the baking sheet. Bake for five minutes.
8. Serve!

Additional Tip:

1. Serve with sauce or mayo.

Spinach and Artichoke Chicken Chaffle

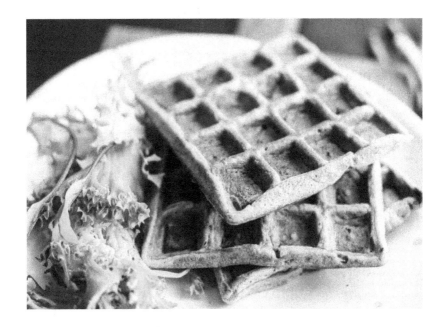

Preparation Time: 3 minutes
Cooking Time: 8 minutes
Serving: 2

Ingredients:

Chicken – 1/3 cup, cooked, diced
Spinach – 1/3 cup, chopped, cooked
Marinated artichokes – 1/3 cup, chopped
Mozzarella cheese – 1/3 cup, shredded
Cream cheese – 1-ounce, softened
Garlic powder – ¼ tsp
Egg – 1

Instructions:

1. Preheat the waffle maker.
2. Mix the mozzarella cheese, cream cheese, garlic powder, and egg into the bowl.
3. Add chicken, artichoke, and spinach and combine well.
4. Pour 1/3 of the batter into the waffle maker. Cook for four minutes.
5. If it is still uncooked, let cook it for two minutes more.

Additional Tip:

1. Serve with ranch dressing.

Corndog Chaffle

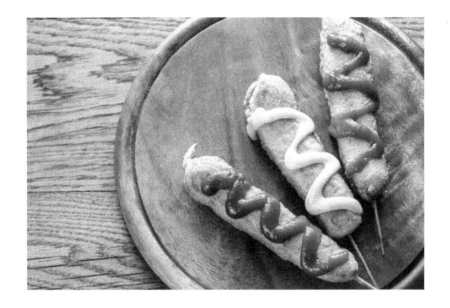

Preparation time: 5 minutes
Cooking time: 5 minutes
Serving: 2

Ingredients:

Flax Egg – combine 1 tbsp ground flaxseed with 3 tbsp of water
Egg – 1
Melted Butter – 1 ½ tbsp
Sweetener granulated – 2 tsp
Almond Flour – 3 tbsp
Baking Powder – ¼ tsp
Egg Yolk – 1
Mexican Blend Cheese – 2 tbsp
Pickled Jalapeños – 1 tbsp, chopped
Cornbread Flavoring – 15-20 drops
Extra cheese – for sprinkling on the waffle maker

Instructions:

1. Preheat the waffle maker.
2. Mix all ingredients into the big bowl. Let sit for five minutes.
3. Add one tbsp water if the mixture is thick.
4. Sprinkle the shredded cheese into the waffle maker.
5. Pour 1/3 of the batter into the iron.
6. Close the lid. Cook for five minutes.
7. When done, remove from the iron.
8. Serve!

Additional Tip:

1. Top with mustard, mayo, and sauce.

Broccoli and Cheese Chaffle

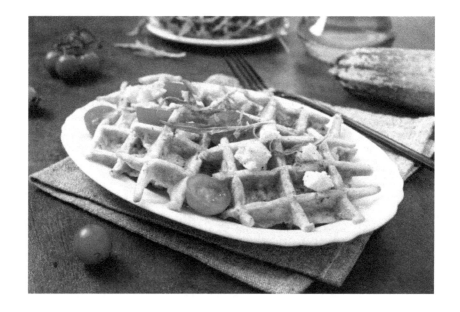

Preparation Time: 2 minutes
Cooking Time: 8 minutes
Servings: 2

Ingredients:

Cheddar cheese – ½ cup
Broccoli – ¼ cup, chopped
Egg – 1
Garlic powder – ¼ tsp
Almond flour – 1 tbsp

Instructions:

1. Preheat the waffle maker.
2. Mix the cheese, egg, garlic powder, and almond flour into the big bowl. Combine well.
3. Pour broccoli and chaffle batter into the waffle maker.
4. Let cook for four minutes.
5. Serve!

Additional Tip:

1. Serve with ranch dressing.

Ham and Cheese Chaffles

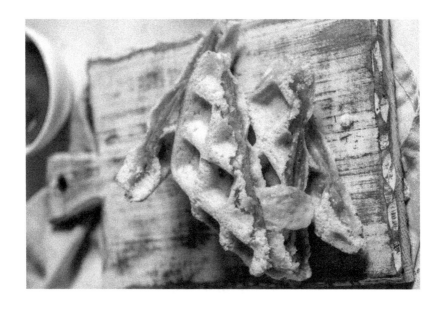

Preparation time: 5 minutes
Cooking time: 6 minutes
Serving: 2

Ingredients:

Egg – 1
Shredded Swiss cheese – ½ cup
Deli ham – ¼ cup, chopped
Garlic salt – ¼ tsp
Mayonnaise – 1 tbsp
Dijon mustard – 2 tsp

Instructions:

1. Preheat the waffle maker.
2. Whisk the eggs into the big bowl.
3. Add Swiss cheese, Deli ham, and garlic salt into the bowl.
4. Mix well. Pour half of the chaffle mixture into the waffle maker.
5. Close the iron. Let cook for three to four minutes.
6. Remove from the waffle maker.
7. Slice chaffle in half and serve!

Additional Tip:

1. Sprinkle with cilantro.

Pulled pork chaffles sandwich

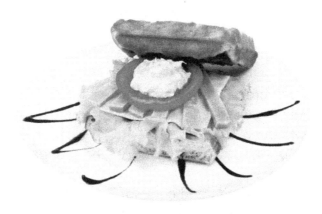

Preparation time: 5 minutes
Cooking time: 28 minutes
Servings: 4

Ingredients:

Eggs – 2, beaten
Cheddar cheese – 1 cup, grated
Baking powder – ¼ tsp
Pork – 2 cup, shredded and cooked
BBQ sauce – 1 tbsp
Shredded coleslaw mix – 2 cups
Apple cider vinegar – 2 tbsp
Salt – ½ tsp
Ranch dressing – ¼ cup

Instructions:

1. First, preheat the waffle maker.
2. Mix the eggs, cheddar cheese, and baking powder into the mixing bowl.
3. Pour half ¼ of the batter into the preheated waffle maker.
4. Close the iron and cook for 7 minutes.
5. Repeat with remaining batter and prepare 4 chaffle.
6. Mix the BBQ sauce and pulled pork into the big bowl. Set it aside.
7. Mix the coleslaw mix, apple cider vinegar, salt, and ranch dressing in another small bowl.
8. Pour the pulled pork on the chaffle.
9. Top with ranch coleslaw and wrap it.
10. Serve!

Additional Tip:

1. Serve with mayo.

Turkey chaffle burger

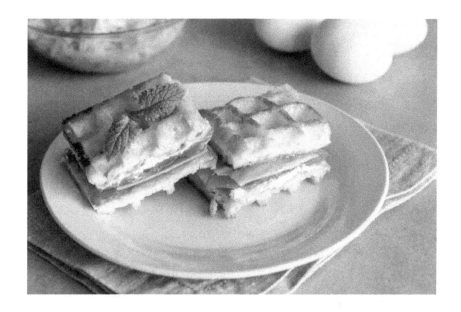

Preparation time: 5 minutes
Cooking time: 10 minutes
Servings: 2

Ingredients:

Ground turkey – 2 cups
Pepper and salt – to taste
Olive oil – 1 tbsp
Romaine lettuce – 1 cup, chopped
Tomato – 1, sliced
Mayonnaise and ketchup – For serving

Garlic chaffles:

Mozzarella cheese – ½ cup, shredded
Cheddar cheese – 1/3 cup
Egg – 1
Garlic powder – 1 tbsp
Italian seasoning – ½ tsp
Baking powder – ¼ tsp

Instructions:

Prepare the garlic chaffle:

2. First, preheat the waffle maker.
3. Add garlic powder, Italian seasoning, egg, and baking powder into the medium bowl and beat well. Add both cheese (mozzarella and cheddar) to the egg mixture and mix well.
4. Add half of the chaffle mixture into the waffle maker. Close the iron.
5. Cook for 2 t0 3 minutes.
6. Meanwhile, combine the ground turkey, salt, and pepper. Prepare the patties from the mixture.
7. Add olive oil to the pan and cook over a medium flame. Add turkey burger and cook on each side.

Additional Tip:

1. Top with mayo.

Lemony fresh herb chaffles

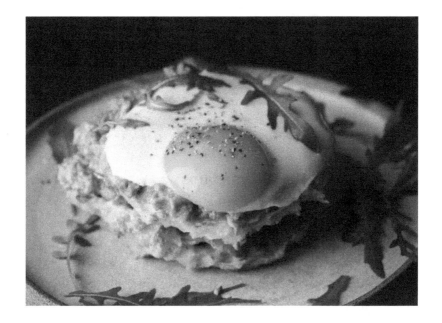

Preparation time: 5 minutes
Cooking time: 24 minutes
Servings: 6

Ingredients:

Ground flaxseed – ½ cup
Eggs – 2
Cheddar cheese – ½ cup, grated
Plain Greek yogurt – 2-4 tbsp
Avocado oil – 1 tbsp
Baking soda – ½ tsp
Fresh lemon juice – 1 tsp
Fresh chives – 2 tbsp, minced
Fresh basil – 1 tbsp, minced
Fresh mint – ½ tbsp, minced
Fresh thyme – ¼ tbsp, minced
Fresh oregano – ¼ tbsp, minced
Ground black pepper and salt – to taste

Instructions:

1. First, preheat the waffle maker.
2. Coat the iron with non-stick cooking spray.
3. Mix all ingredients into the big bowl.
4. Pour one portion of the batter into the waffle maker.
5. Let cook for four minutes. Repeat with remaining mixture.
6. Serve!

Additional Tip:

1. Garnish with lemon wedge.

Ingredients:

Egg – 1
Pork panko – ¼ cup
Mozzarella cheese – ½ cup
Pickle juice – 1 tbsp
Thin pickle slices – 6-8

Instructions:

1. Preheat the waffle maker.
2. Mix all ingredients into the bowl.
3. Place pickle slice and then add thin layer of mixture.
4. Pour into the waffle maker. Close the iron.
5. Cook for four minutes.
6. Serve!

Additional Tip:

1. Serve with ketchup.

Turnip hash brown chaffles

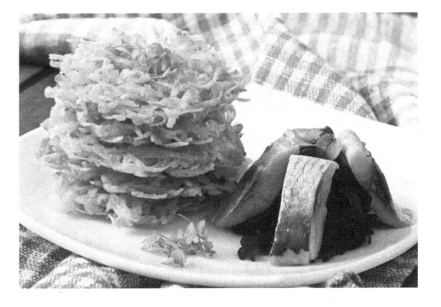

Preparation time: 10 minutes
Cooking time: 40 minutes
Servings: 6

Ingredients:

Turnip – 1, shredded and peeled
White onion – ½, minced
Garlic cloves – 2, crushed
Gouda cheese – 1 cup, grated
Eggs – 2, beaten
Ground black pepper and salt – to taste

Instructions:

1. Preheat the waffle maker.
2. Add turnips into the oven-safe bowl. Add one tbsp water and place into the oven and cook for 1 to 2 minutes.
3. Transfer the mixture to the bowl and then add remaining ingredients except Gouda cheese.
4. Add 3 tbsp of mixture into the waffle maker.
5. Cook for 5 minutes.
6. Serve!

Additional Tip:

1. Sprinkle with black pepper.

Fried Pickle Chaffle Sticks

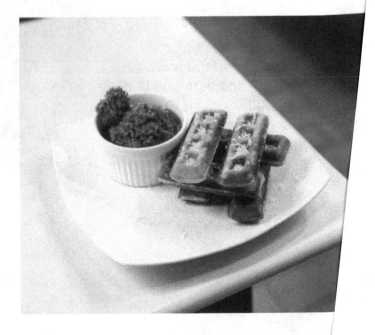

Preparation time: 5 minu
Cooking time: 4 minute
Servings: 2

Sloppy joe chaffle

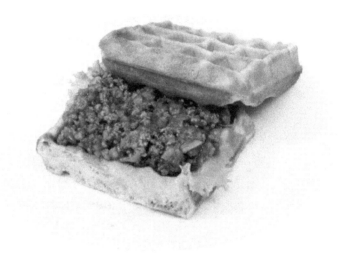

Preparation time: 5 minutes
Cooking time: 4 minutes
Servings: 2

Ingredients:

Sloppy Joe ingredients:

Ground beef – 1 lb
Onion powder – 1 tsp
Garlic – 1 tsp, minced
Tomato paste – 3 tbsp
Salt – ½ tsp
Pepper – ¼ tsp
Chili powder – 1 tbsp
Cocoa powder – 1 tsp
Bone broth beef – ½ cup
Soy sauce – 1 tsp
Mustard powder – 1 tsp
Swerve brown – 1 tsp
Paprika – ½ tsp

Cornbread chaffle ingredients:

Egg – 1
Cheddar cheese – ½ cup
Jalapeno – 5 slices, diced
Red hot sauce – 1 tsp
Corn extract – ¼ tsp
Pinch salt

Instructions:

1. Preheat the waffle maker.
2. Mix ground beef with pepper and salt. Add remaining ingredients and combine well. Let simmer the mixture.
3. Whip the egg into the bowl and then add remaining ingredient for chaffle.
4. Coat the waffle maker with non-stick cooking spray.
5. Pour half of the mixture into the waffle maker.
6. Cook for flour minutes.
7. Add warm sloppy Joe mix onto the chaffle and serve!

Additional Tip:

1. Sprinkle with fresh cilantro.

Keto Sausage Ball Chaffle

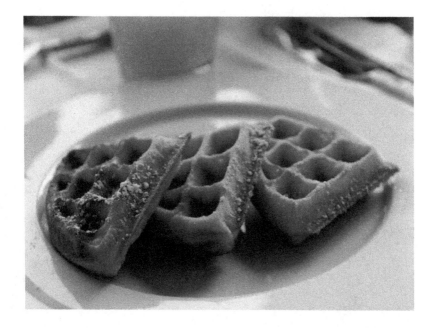

Preparation time: 5 minutes
Cooking time: 4 minutes
Servings: 2

Ingredients:

Italian sausage – 1 pound
Almond flour – 1 cup
Baking powder – 2 tsp
Sharp cheddar cheese – 1 cup, shredded
Parmesan cheese – ¼ cup, grated
Egg – 1

Instructions:

1. Preheat the waffle maker.
2. Mix all ingredients into the big mixing bowl.
3. Place the paper towel under the waffle maker.
4. Add three tbsp of the batter into the waffle maker.
5. Cook for three minutes. Flip over and cook for two minutes.
6. Serve!

Additional Tip:

1. Serve with mayo.

Baked Potato Chaffle

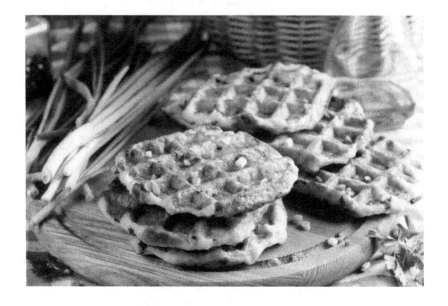

Preparation time: 5 minutes
Cooking time: 15 minutes
Servings: 2

Ingredients:

Jicama root – 1
Onion – 1/2, minced
Garlic cloves – 1, pressed
Halloumi cheese – 1 cup
Eggs – 2, whisked
Salt and pepper – as needed

Instructions:

1. First, peel jicama and add into the food processor.
2. Add shredded jicama into the colander. Sprinkle with one to two tsp salt. Combine well. Drain it. Microwave it for five to eight minutes.
3. Preheat the waffle maker. Sprinkle cheese into the waffle maker.
4. Add three tbsp of the mixture into the waffle maker. Top with cheese.
5. Let cook for five minutes. Turnover and cook for two minutes more.

Additional Tip:

1. Top with bacon, cheese, chives, and jicama, sour cream.

Okra Fritter Chaffles

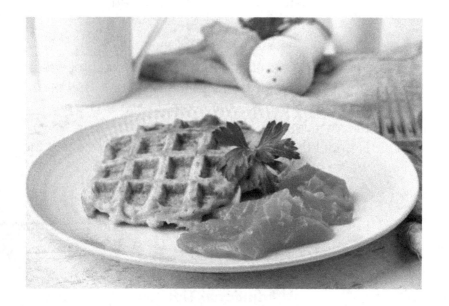

Preparation time: 5 minutes
Cooking time: 7 minutes
Servings: 2

Ingredients:

Egg – 1
Mayo – 1 tbsp
Heavy cream – 2 tbsp
Seasoning – ½ tbsp
Onion powder
Salt and pepper – to taste
Almond flour – ¼ cup
Okra fresh or frozen – 1 cup, thawed
Mozzarella cheese – ¼ cup, shredded

Instructions:

1. Preheat the waffle maker.
2. Whip the seasoning, heavy cream, mayo, and egg into the bowl.
3. Let rest for few minutes. Add in okra and combine well.
4. Pour three tbsp of the batter into the waffle maker.
5. Cook for five minutes. Flip over and cook for two minutes more.

Additional Tip:

1. Sprinkle with sea salt.

Avocado Toast Chaffle

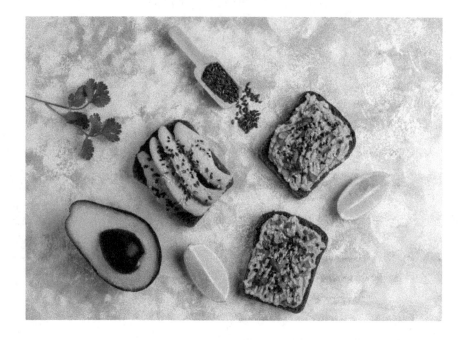

Preparation time: 5 minutes
Cooking time: 4 minutes
Servings: 2

Ingredients:

Mozzarella cheese – ½ cup, shredded
Egg – 1
Pinch of salt
Avocado – 1/2, mashed

Instructions:

1. Preheat the waffle maker.
2. Whip the egg into the bowl. Add rest of ingredients and combine well.
3. Pour half of the batter into the preheated waffle maker.
4. Cook for four minutes.
5. Serve!

Additional Tip:

1. Serve with butter.

Yummy Chili chaffle

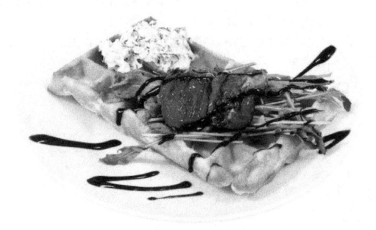

Preparation time: 5 minutes
Cooking time: 7-9 minutes
Servings: 4

Ingredients:

Eggs – 4
Parmesan cheese – ½ cup, grated
Cheddar cheese – 1 ½ cup, yellow
Red chili pepper – 1
Pepper and salt – to taste
Dried garlic powder – ½ tsp
Dried basil – 1 tsp
Almond flour – 2 tbsp
Olive oil – 2 tbsp, for brushing

Instructions:

1. Preheat the waffle maker.
2. Break eggs into the medium bowl. Add cheddar cheese and parmesan cheese into the bowl.
3. Combine well. After that, add chopped chili pepper – season with dried basil, dried garlic powder, pepper, and salt.
4. Next, brush the waffle maker with olive oil.
5. Pour mixture into the waffle iron.
6. Close the iron. Cook for seven to eight minutes until golden brown.
7. Serve!

Additional Tip:

1. Serve with chili sauce.

Tasty Bacon chaffles

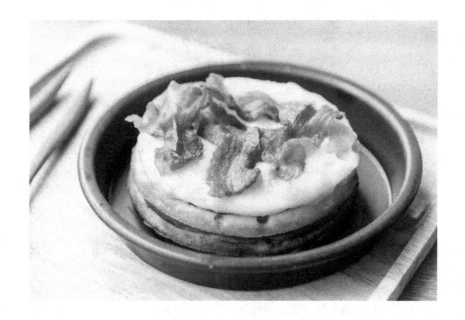

Preparation time: 5 minutes
Cooking time: 7-9 minutes
Servings: 4

Ingredients:

Eggs – 4
Shredded mozzarella cheese – 2 cups
Chopped bacon – 2-ounce
Pepper and salt – to taste
Dried oregano – 1 tsp
Olive oil – 2 tbsp, for brushing

Instructions:

1. Preheat the waffle maker.
2. Break eggs into the big bowl. Add mozzarella cheese. Combine well.
3. Add in chopped bacon – season with dried oregano, pepper, and salt.
4. Brush the waffle maker with olive oil.
5. Pour mixture into the waffle maker. Close the iron.
6. Cook for seven to eight minutes.
7. Serve!

Additional Tip:

1. Serve with mayo and sauce.

Crispy fish and chaffle bites

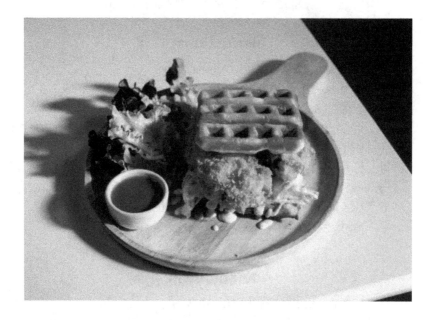

Preparation time: 5 minutes
Cooking time: 15 minutes
Servings: 4

Ingredients:

Cod fillets – 1 lb, cut into four pieces
Sea salt – 1 tsp
Garlic powder – 1 tsp
Egg – 1, whisked
Almond flour – 1 cup
Avocado oil – 2 tbsp

Chaffle ingredients:

Eggs – 2
Cheddar cheese – ½ cup
Almond flour – 2 tbsp
Italian seasoning – ½ tsp

Instructions:

1. Combine chaffle ingredients into the medium bowl. Prepare four squares.
2. Add the mixture into the waffle maker.
3. Meanwhile, combine the garlic powder, pepper, and salt into the mixing bowl. Immerse the cod fillets into the mixture and then dip in almond flour.
4. Add oil into the skillet and then add fish cubes and cook for two to three minutes.
5. Serve over chaffles.

Additional Tip:

1. Serve with sauce.

Chicken zinger chaffle

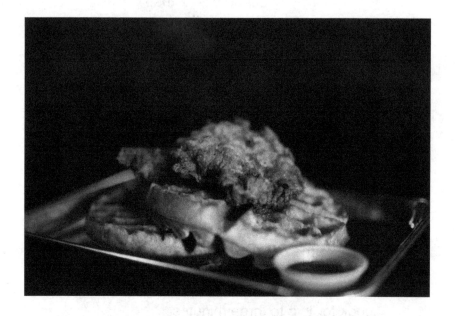

Preparation time: 5 minutes
Cooking time: 15 minutes
Servings: 2

Ingredients:

Chicken breast – 1, cut into two pieces
Coconut flour – ½ cup
Grated parmesan cheese – ¼ cup
Paprika – 1 tsp
Garlic powder – ½ tsp
Onion powder – ½ tsp
Egg – 1, beaten
Avocado oil – for frying
Lettuce leaves – as needed
BBQ sauce

Chaffle ingredients:

Baking powder – 1 tsp
Almond flour – ¼ cup
Eggs – 2
Cheese – 4-ounce

Instructions:

1. Preheat the waffle maker.
2. Combine chaffle ingredients into the big bowl.
3. Pour chaffle mixture into the preheated waffle maker.
4. Cook for two minutes.
5. Meanwhile, combine the pepper, salt, onion powder, garlic powder, paprika, parmesan cheese, and coconut flour into the medium bowl.
6. Immerse the chicken in the coconut flour mixture and then whisked egg.
7. Add avocado oil into the medium skillet and add chicken and cook on each side.
8. Keep chicken zinger between two warm chaffle. Top with lettuce leaves and BBQ sauce.
9. Serve!

Additional Tip:

1. Serve with BBQ sauce.

Bruscetta chaffle

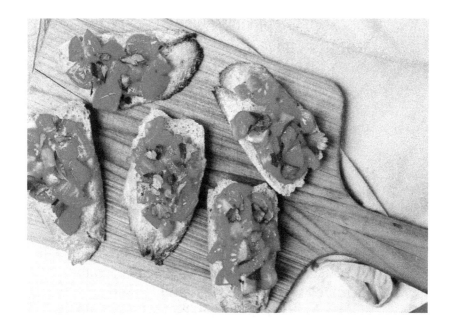

Preparation time: 5 minutes
Cooking time: 5 minutes
Servings: 2

Ingredients:

Marinara sauce – 2 tbsp, sugar-free
Mozzarella cheese – 2 tbsp, shredded
Olives – 1 tbsp, sliced
Tomato – 1, sliced
Pesto sauce – 1 tbsp
Basil leaves

Chaffle ingredients:

Baking powder – 1 tsp
Almond flour – ¼ cup
Eggs – 2
Cheese – 4-ounce

Instructions:

1. Preheat the waffle maker.
2. Mix all ingredients for chaffle.
3. Add chaffle mixture into the waffle maker. Cook for two minutes.
4. Meanwhile, scatter marinara sauce on the chaffle.
5. Add pesto on the marinara sauce. Top with mozzarella cheese, olives, and tomato.
6. Place into the oven and bake for three minutes.

Additional Tip:

1. Garnish with fresh basil.

Okonomiyaki Chaffle

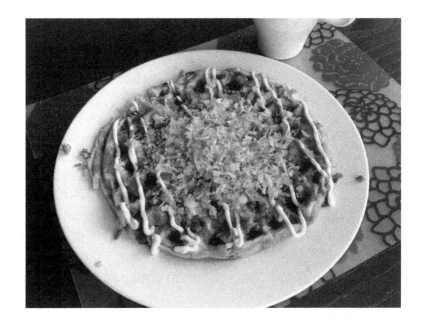

Preparation time: 8 minutes
Cooking time: 15 minutes
Serving: 1

Ingredients:

Batter:

Eggs – 2, beaten
Cheddar cheese – 1/3 cup, shredded
Cabbage leaves – 2, chopped
Ham – 1 slice, chopped
Spring onions – 1 bunch, green parts chopped
Salt – 1 pinch
White pepper – 1 dash
Avocado oil

Topping:

Japanese mayonnaise
Bulldog tonkatsu sauce
A handful of bonito flakes

Instructions:

1. Preheat the waffle maker.
2. Coat the waffle iron with avocado oil.
3. Add egg, cabbage, ham, and cheese into the bowl and beat well. Add one tbsp chopped spring onion. Combine well.
4. Pour mixture into the waffle maker.
5. Cook for five minutes.
6. When cooked, remove from the waffle maker.
7. Add one tbsp of chopped spring onion onto the chaffle.

Additional Tip:

1. Top with Japanese mayonnaise, Bulldog tonkatsu sauce, and bonito flakes.

Crab cake chaffle

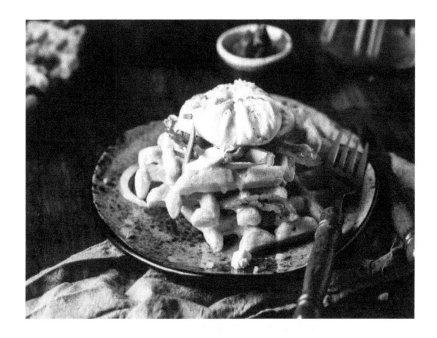

Preparation time: 8 minutes
Cooking time: 5 minutes
Serving: 2

Ingredients:

1/4 cup shredded mozzarella – ¼ cup
Almond flour – 1 tbsp
Nutritional yeast – 1 tsp
Old bay seasoning – ¼ tsp
Fresh black pepper – 3-4, ground
Egg – 1
Red pepper – 1 tbsp, diced
Celery – 1 tbsp, diced
Onion – 1 tbsp, diced
Garlic – ¼ tsp, minced
Lump crab meat – 2-ounce

Instructions:

1. Add black pepper, old bay seasoning, nutritional yeast, almond flour, and mozzarella cheese into the blender or food processor.
2. Pulse for eight times until mixture is look like a bread crumbs.
3. Add egg to the dry mixture and blend for five seconds.
4. Place the batter into the mixing bowl. Add crab meat, garlic, onion, celery, and red pepper. Combine with spatula.
5. Pour half of the batter into the waffle maker. Cook for four to five minutes.
6. When done, cool it for two to three minutes.
7. Serve!

Additional Tip:

1. Serve with sauce.

Roast Beef Chaffle Sandwich

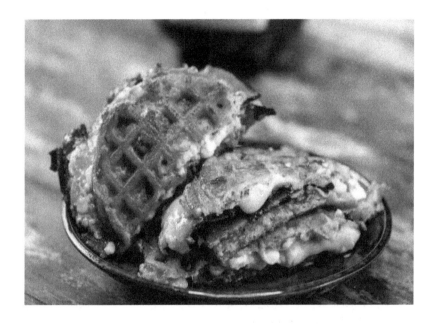

Preparation time: 8 minutes
Cooking time: 5 minutes
Serving: 2

Ingredients:

Chaffle bread ingredients:

Mozzarella cheese – ½ cup, shredded
Egg – 1
Onion powder – ¼ tsp
Garlic powder – ¼ tsp

Sandwich ingredients:

Provolone cheese – thickly slice
Cheddar cheese – 1 slice
Mayo – 1 tbsp
Dijon mustard – 1 tsp

Instructions:

Roast beef chaffle sandwich instructions:

1. Preheat the waffle maker.
2. Whip the egg into the bowl.
3. Add egg, seasonings, and cheese in to the bowl. Combine well.
4. Pour half of batter into the waffle maker.
5. Cook for four minutes.
6. Meanwhile, add roasted beef, Dijon mustard, mayo, and cheese on the sandwich.
7. Add one tsp butter into the frying pan and add prepared chaffle sandwich into the pan and cook for two to three minutes.
8. Serve!

Additional Tip:

1. Sprinkle with cilantro.

Buffalo hummus beef chaffle

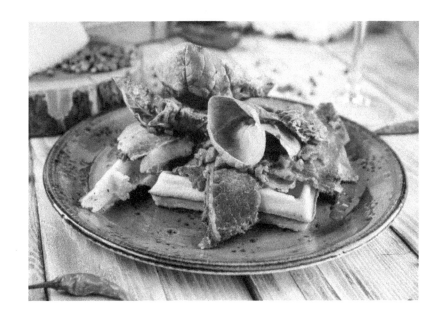

Preparation time: 10 minutes
Cooking time: 32 minutes
Servings: 2

Ingredients:

Celery stalks – 2, chopped
Hummus – 3 tbsp
Buffalo sauce – ¼ cup
Chicken breast – 2, diced and cooked
Ground black pepper and salt – to taste
Scallions – 2, chopped
Cheddar cheese – 1 ¼ cup, grated
Eggs – 2
Crumbled blue cheese – ¼ cup, for topping

Instructions:

1. First, preheat the waffle maker.
2. Mix the one cup of cheddar cheese, egg, scallions, salt, and black pepper into the medium bowl.
3. Pour half of batter into the waffle maker. Close the iron.
4. Cook for 7 minutes.
5. Preheat the oven to 400 degrees F.
6. Next, line the baking sheet with parchment paper.
7. Cut chaffle into pieces and place on the baking sheet.
8. Mix the chicken with buffalo sauce, hummus, and celery into the bowl.
9. Add chicken mixture into the chaffles and top with remaining cheddar cheese and place on the baking sheet and bake for 4 minutes and serve!

Additional Tip:

1. Serve with ketchup.

Kale Chaffle

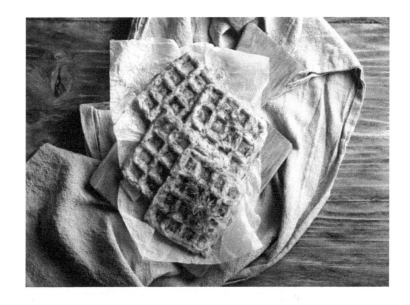

Preparation time: 30 minutes
Cooking time: 5 minutes
Servings: 2

Ingredients:

For the chaffle:

Kale – 9-ounce
Salt – to taste
Soft butter – 6-ounce
Eggs – 4
One pinch of salt
Pastry flour – 9-ounce
Milk – 9-ounce
Freshly ground peppers – as needed
Nutmeg – as needed
Vegetable oil – as needed

For the sauce:

Whipped cream – 7-ounce
Yogurt – 3-ounce
Dill weed – 2 tbsp, chopped
Lemon juice and salt – as needed

Instructions:

1. Preheat the waffle maker.
2. Wash the kale under clean water. Next, blanch in the salted boiling water for 5 minutes.
3. Drain it and wash under cold water. Chop them,
4. Add egg into the bowl and beat well. Sprinkle with salt and flour.
5. Next, add milk and kale and combine well.
6. Let sit for 30 minutes.
7. Season with pepper, salt, and nutmeg.
8. Coat the waffle maker with oil. Pour batter into the waffle maker.
9. Cook for five minutes.
10. For sauce: Mix the yogurt and dill into the bowl – season with salt and lemon juice.
11. Serve over chaffle.

Additional Tip:

1. Serve with mayo.

Keto Chaffle Taco Shells

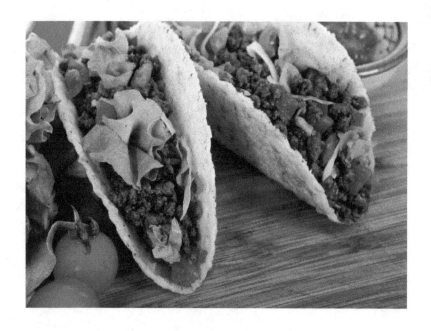

Preparation Time: 5 minutes
Cooking Time: 20 minutes
Servings: 5

Ingredients:

Almond flour – 1 tbsp
Taco blend cheese – 1 cup
Eggs – 2
Taco seasoning – ¼ tsp

Instructions:

1. Combine the taco seasoning, eggs, taco blend cheese, and almond flour into the bowl. Combine well.
2. Add one and half tbsp of the taco chaffle batter into the waffle maker.
3. Cook for four minutes.
4. Serve!

Additional Tip:

1. Serve with mayo.

French dip chaffle sandwich keto

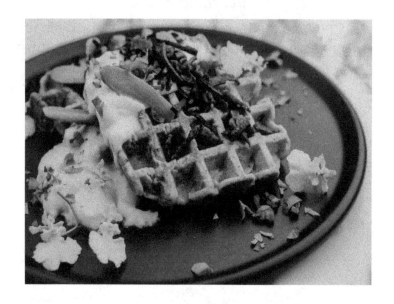

Preparation Time: 5 minutes
Cooking Time: 12 minutes
Servings: 2

Ingredients:

Egg white – 1
Mozzarella cheese – ¼ cup, shredded
Sharp cheddar cheese – ¼ cup, shredded
Water – ¾ tsp
Coconut flour – 1 tsp
Baking powder – ¼ tsp
Pinch of salt

Instructions:

1. Preheat the waffle maker. Grease the waffle maker with oil.
2. Preheat the oven to 425 degrees Fahrenheit.
3. Mix all ingredients into the bowl. Stir well.
4. Add half of the batter into the waffle maker. Close the lid.
5. Cook for four minutes.
6. When cooked, remove the chaffle from the waffle maker.
7. Place chaffle on the baking sheet lined with parchment paper.
8. Add 1/3 cup of keto roast beef on the top of chaffle. Add a slice of shredded or deli cheese.
9. Place into the oven and bake for five minutes. Turn to broiler and broil for one minute.

Additional Tip:

1. Serve with dipping sauce.

Egg & cheese hash browns chaffle

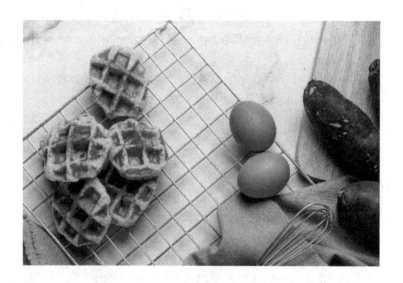

Preparation time: 5 minutes
Cooking time: 6 minutes
Servings: 4-5

Ingredients:

20-ounce simply potatoes hash browns – shredded
Eggs – 3
Milk – ¼ cup
Shredded sharp cheddar cheese – 1 cup
1/4 cup fresh chives – for garnishing, chopped
Salt and pepper – to taste
Sour cream – for serving, if desired

Instructions:

1. Preheat the waffle iron over a medium-high flame.
2. Spray the waffle iron with non-stick cooking spray.
3. Whisk the milk and eggs into the mixing bowl.
4. Add in chives, cheese, and potatoes – season with pepper and salt.
5. Add half of the batter into the waffle maker. Cook for five minutes.
6. Serve!

Additional Tip:

1. Serve with butter.

Big Mac Chaffle

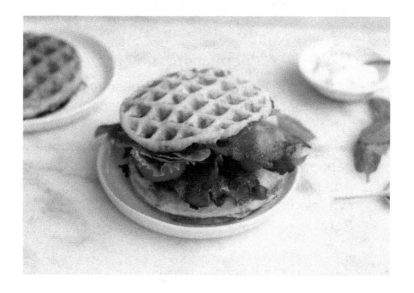

Preparation time: 10 minutes
Cooking time: 10 minutes
Serving: 1

Ingredients:

For the cheeseburgers:

Ground beef – 1/3 pound
Garlic salt – ½ tsp
American cheese – 2 slices

For the Chaffles:

Egg – 1
Shredded mozzarella cheese – ½ cup
Garlic salt – ¼ tsp

For the Big Mac Sauce:

Mayonnaise – 2 tsp
Ketchup – 1 tsp
Dill pickle relish – 1 tsp
Splash vinegar – to taste

To assemble:

Shredded lettuce – 2 tbsp
Dill pickles – 3-4
Onion – 2 tsp, minced

Instructions:

To make the burgers:

1. Heat the griddle over a medium-high flame.
2. Split the ground beef into two-sized balls.
3. Place on the griddle and cook for one minute.
4. Sprinkle with garlic salt. Cook for two minutes more.
5. Flip over and sprinkle with remaining garlic salt.
6. Cook for two minutes. Add one slice of cheese over each patty.
7. Stack the patties and keep them on the plate. Cover with foil.

To make the chaffles:

1. Preheat the waffle iron. Coat with non-stick spray.
2. Whisk the garlic salt, cheese, and egg and mix well.

3. Add half of the egg mixture to the waffle maker.
4. Cook for two to three minutes.

To make the Big Mac Sauce:

1. Whisk all ingredients.

To assemble burgers:

1. Top chaffle with onion, pickles, shredded lettuce, burger patties.
2. Scatter the big Mac sauce on the chaffle and add sauce over the sandwich.

Additional Tip:

1. Serve with mayo and sauce.

Keto Whoopie Chaffle

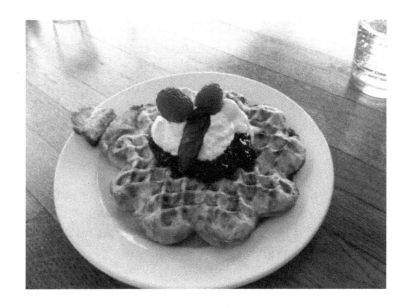

Preparation time: 10 minutes
Cooking time: 10 minutes
Serving: 1

Ingredients:

Egg – 1
Cream cheese – 1-ounce, softened
Vanilla – ½ tsp
Monkfruit or erithrytol – 1 tbsp
Cocoa powder – 1 ½ tsp
Baking powder – ¼ tsp

Filling:

Cream cheese – 3-ounce
Heavy cream – 2 tbsp
Liquid stevia – 12-15 drops
Vanilla – ½ tsp

Instructions:

1. Preheat the waffle maker.
2. Whisk the cream cheese and egg into the bowl. Add remaining ingredients and whisk it well.
3. Pour the mixture into the waffle iron and cook for six to eight minutes.
4. Let cool it.

For filling:

1. Combine all ingredients using a hand mixer. Scatter between two chaffles and place them into the refrigerator for ten to fifteen minutes.

Additional Tip:

1. Top with cream cheese.

Garlic chicken alfredo chaffle pizza

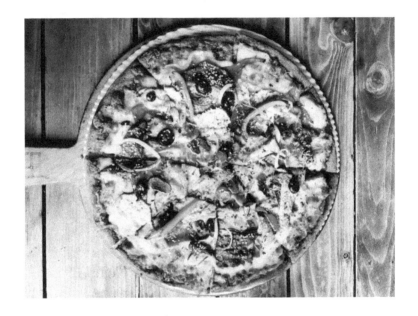

Preparation Time: 5 minutes
Cooking Time: 20 minutes
Servings: 5

Ingredients:

For the chaffles:

Coconut flour – ¾ cup
Italian seasoning – 1 tsp
Onion powder – 1 tsp
Garlic powder – ½ tsp
Baking powder – ½ tsp
Sea salt – ½ tsp
Eggs – six
Grass fed butter – ¼ cup, melted
Almond milk or coconut milk – 1 ½ cups
Parmesan cheese – ½ cup, shredded

For the garlic parmesan cream sauce:

Heavy cream – ¾ cup
Parmesan cheese – ¾ cup, grated
Cloves garlic – 3, minced
Sea salt – to taste
Cracked black pepper

For the pizza toppings:

Mozzarella cheese – 1 ¼ cup, shredded
Chicken – 1 lb, cooked and cubed
Thick sliced bacon – 10 strips, cooked and crumbled
Mushrooms – 3, thinly sliced
Red onion – couple slices, thinly sliced
Chives – 2, chopped

Instructions:

For the chaffle:

1. Mix the sea salt, baking powder, garlic powder, onion powder, Italian seasoning, and coconut flour into the mixing bowl.
2. Break eggs in another bowl. Whisk with coconut milk and melted butter.
3. Add egg mixture into the dry ingredients.

4. Fold the parmesan cheese into the mixture using a rubber spatula.
5. Preheat the waffle maker. Pour the batter into the waffle maker.
6. Cook until crispy.

For the garlic parmesan cream sauce:

1. Add crack black pepper, sea salt, garlic, parmesan cheese, and heavy cream to the saucepan and cook over a medium-high flame.
2. Boil it and then decrease the speed of the flame to low. Stir and simmer until thick.

For the chaffle pizzas:

1. Preheat the oven to 350 degrees Fahrenheit.
2. Top chaffle with garlic-parmesan cream sauce, and then cover the sauce with mozzarella cheese.
3. Top with red onion, mushrooms, bacon, and chicken.
4. Place into the oven and bake for seventeen minutes.

Additional Tip:

1. Top with chives.
2. Serve with sauce.

Vegan keto chaffle

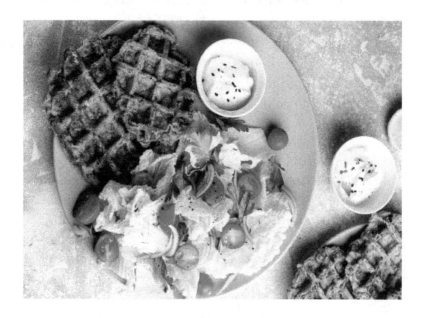

Preparation Time: 5 minutes
Cooking Time: 20 minutes
Servings: 5

Ingredients:

Flaxseed meal – 1 tbsp
Water – 2 ½ tbsp
Low-carb vegan cheese – ¼ cup
Coconut flour – 2 tbsp
Vegan cream cheese – 1 tbsp, softened
Pinch of salt

Instructions:

1. Preheat the waffle maker over a medium-high flame.
2. Combine water and flaxseed meal into the bowl. Let rest for five minutes until thick.
3. Whisk all ingredients for vegan chaffle.
4. Pour half of the batter into the waffle maker. Close the iron.
5. Let cook for three to five minutes.
6. Serve!

Additional Tip:

1. Top with fresh chives.

Rosemary olive Focaccia Chaffles

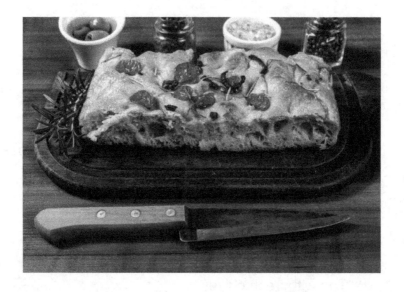

Preparation time: 5 minutes
Cooking time: 10 minutes
Serving: 2

Ingredients:

Savory chaffles:

Egg – 1
Mozzarella cheese – ½ cup
Almond flour – ¼ cup
Baking powder – ¼ tsp

Chaffles filling:

Egg white – 1
Mozzarella cheese – ½ cup, grated
Extra-virgin olive oil – 1 tsp
Almond flour – 2 tbsp
Parmesan cheese – 2 tbsp, grated
Baking powder – ¼ tsp
Pinch of black pepper
Dried rosemary – ¼ tsp
Black, green, or kalamata olives – 6, sliced

Topping:

Extra-virgin olive oil – 1 tbsp
Garlic – ¼ tsp, minced

Instructions:

For chaffle filling:

1. Mix the one tsp olive oil, egg white, and mozzarella cheese into the blender. Blend it.
2. Add parmesan cheese, baking powder, and black pepper and blend again.
3. Add rosemary and olives and stir well.

For making savory chaffles:

1. Preheat the waffle maker. Coat the waffle maker with non-stick cooking spray.
2. Pour all savory ingredients into the bowl. Mix well.
3. Add into the food processor and blend well.
4. Pour half of the batter into the waffle maker.

5. Close the iron. Cook for 3 to 4 minutes.
6. During this, mix the olive oil and minced garlic and prepare the topping.
7. Let cool it. Drizzle with garlic-olive mixture over the chaffle.

Additional Tip:

1. Sprinkle with fresh parsley.

Keto Reuben Chaffle Sandwich

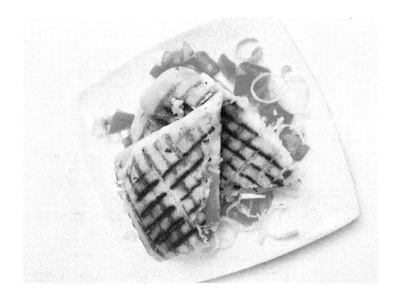

Preparation time: 5 minutes
Cooking time: 8 minutes
Servings: 1

Ingredients:

Egg – 1
Mozzarella cheese – ½ cup
Almond flour – 2 tbsp
Low-carb Thousand Island dressing – 2 tbsp
Baking powder – ¼ tsp
Caraway seeds – ¼ tsp
Corned beef – 2 slices
Swiss cheese – 1 slice
Sauerkraut – 2 tbsp

Instructions:

1. Preheat the waffle maker.
2. Whisk the egg, mozzarella cheese, almond flour, one tbsp Thousand Island dressing, caraway seeds, and baking powder into the bowl.
3. After that, add the Reuben mixture into the waffle maker.
4. Close the iron. Cook for 5 to 7 minutes.
5. Add corned beef over the parchment paper.
6. Top with Swiss cheese.
7. Place into the oven and bake for 20 to 30 seconds.
8. Remove from the oven.
9. Spread Thousand Island dressing over the chaffle.
10. Next, a layer of Swiss cheese and corned beef.

Additional Tip:

1. Top with sauerkraut.

Keto Tuna Melt Chaffle

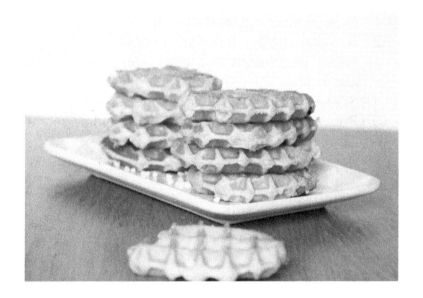

Preparation time: 5 minutes
Cooking time: 8 minutes
Serving: 2

Ingredients:

Tuna with no water – 2.6-ounce
Mozzarella cheese – ½ cup
Egg – 1
Pinch of salt

Instructions:

1. First, preheat the waffle maker.
2. Beat the egg into the medium bowl.
3. Add tuna, mozzarella cheese, and salt into the bowl. Mix well.
4. Sprinkle with cheese into the waffle maker.
5. Pour the batter into the waffle iron and close the lid.
6. Cook for four minutes.
7. Serve!

Additional Tip:

1. Serve with mayonnaise.

Keto parmesan garlic chaffles

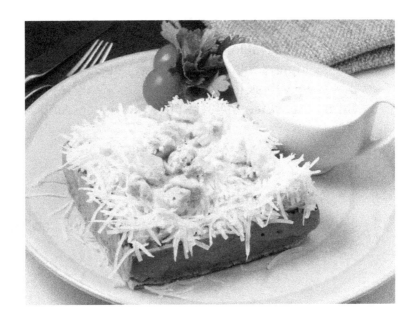

Preparation Time: 2 minutes
Cooking Time: 4 minutes
Servings: 2

Ingredients:

Shredded mozzarella cheese – ½ cup
Whole egg – 1, beaten
Grated parmesan cheese – ¼ cup
Italian seasoning – 1 tsp
Garlic powder – ¼ tsp

Instructions:

1. Preheat the waffle maker.
2. Mix all ingredients except mozzarella cheese into the bowl. Whisk it well.
3. Spray the waffle maker with non-stick cooking spray.
4. Pour half of the batter into the waffle maker.
5. Cook for three to five minutes.

Additional Tip:

1. Serve with grated parmesan cheese, basil, chopped parsley, and drizzle with olive oil.

Keto chaffle calzone

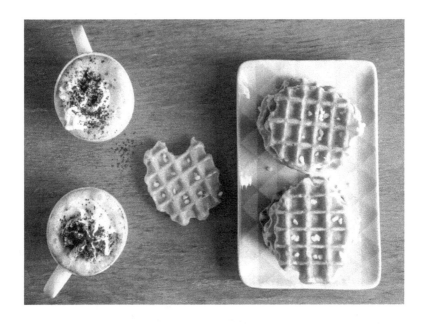

Preparation Time: 15 minutes
Cooking Time: 10 minutes
Servings: 4

Ingredients:
Chaffle Batter:
Eggs – 2
Mozzarella cheese – 1-1/4 cups, grated
Parmesan cheese – ¼ cup
Coconut flour – 4 tsp
Butter – 1 tbsp, melted
Psyllium husk powder – 1 tsp
Baking soda – ½ tsp, sifted
Fillings and Assemble:
Link sausage – 1, big, sliced, or Bulk sausage fried up – ½ cup
Mozzarella cheese – 1 cup, grated, cut in half
Vegetable pizza toppings:
artichoke hearts, mushrooms,
sliced onions, olives – 2/3 cup
Marinara sauce – 2 tbsp

Instructions:
1. Preheat the waffle maker.
2. Preheat the oven to 350 degrees F.
3. Mix all chaffle ingredients: baking soda, psyllium husk powder, almond flour or coconut, parmesan cheese, mozzarella cheese, and eggs into the mixing bowl.
4. Add batter into the waffle maker.
5. Cook for two minutes. Transfer the cooked chaffle to the baking sheet.
6. Spread half of the marinara and top with sausage and cheese.
7. Add cheese and pizza veggies over it.
8. Fold the chaffle and seal the edges.
9. Place on the baking sheet. Place into the oven and bake for eight to ten minutes.
10. Serve!

Additional Tip:

1. Sprinkle with fresh chives.

Conclusion

This cookbook is the work of many passionate souls who loves chaffles. I created simple, delicious, and healthy recipes for you. Most importantly, each recipe has a stock-free image that will guide you. I want to say thank you to all readers who choose this cookbook. It is a big honor for me.

Notes